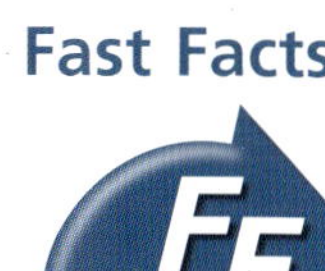

Fast Facts: Rheumatology Highlights 2005–06

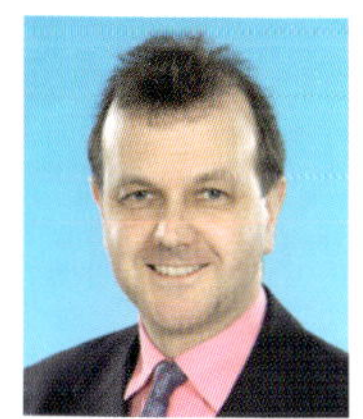

Edited by John D Isaacs PhD FRCP
Professor of Clinical Rheumatology
University of Newcastle upon Tyne, UK

HEALTH PRESS

Fast Facts: Rheumatology Highlights 2005–06
First published March 2006

Health Press Limited, Elizabeth House, Queen Street, Abingdon,
Oxford OX14 3LN, UK
Tel: +44 (0)1235 523233
Fax: +44 (0)1235 523238

Book orders can be placed by telephone or via the website.
For regional distributors or to order via the website, please go to:
www.fastfacts.com
For telephone orders, please call 01752 202301 (UK), +44 1752 202301 (Europe),
1 800 247 6553 (USA, toll free) or +1 419 281 1802 (Americas).

A CIP record for this title is available from the British Library.

ISBN 1-903734-86-X

Isaacs, JD (John)
Fast Facts: Rheumatology Highlights 2005–06/
John D Isaacs

Typesetting and page layout by Zed, Oxford, UK.
Printed by Fine Print (Services) Ltd, Oxford, UK.

Printed with vegetable inks on fully biodegradable and recyclable paper manufactured from sustainable forests.

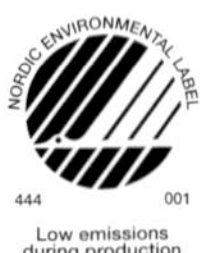

Low emissions during production

Low chlorine

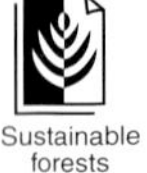
Sustainable forests

Introduction

The practice of rheumatology continues to undergo rapid change. On the epidemiological front it has become clear that rheumatoid arthritis (RA) has a long preclinical phase, characterized by the presence of autoantibodies and subclinical inflammation (page 24). In the future this may provide an opportunity for pre-emptive treatment, as is starting to happen in other autoimmune diseases.

From a genetic perspective, we are finally beginning to discover genes outside of the human leukocyte antigen (HLA) complex that are linked to and associated with RA (page 30). Some of these show similar associations with other autoimmune diseases, suggesting fundamental defects of immune regulation, and perhaps underlying the familial propensity to autoimmunity that can affect different organ systems.

Immune regulation is also becoming an important theme in the therapy of autoimmunity. B-cell depletion is proving highly effective in the treatment of RA and other inflammatory conditions (page 37). Similarly, there is now evidence that autologous stem-cell transplantation may unleash powerful immunoregulatory mechanisms, at least in some conditions (page 74). Some of these mechanisms are underpinned by the existence of regulatory lymphocyte subsets. Our understanding of these cells is increasing exponentially, suggesting regimens that may harness their powerful effects for patient benefit (page 98). Cytokine blockade continues to be a popular approach for the treatment of RA that is refractory to standard therapy, and interleukin-15 appears to be a promising target (page 47).

Despite these advances, most of our patients still need symptomatic treatment, and the association of cyclooxygenase-2 (COX-2) antagonism with cardiovascular disease has significantly limited our therapeutic options. The jury is still out on the implications of these discoveries and, indeed, their relevance to conventional non-steroidal anti-inflammatory drugs (NSAIDs). The chapter on the risks and benefits of COX-2 inhibitors (page 15) provides a well-balanced and up-to-date summary of this area.

Meanwhile, as treatments for RA improve, and particularly whilst the safety of NSAIDs remains unresolved, osteoarthritis is set to become our major challenge as rheumatologists. The opening chapter of this book provides a state-of-the-art summary of current osteoarthritis therapies (page 7).

Stem cells and tissue engineering have assumed prominence across the entire spectrum of medical specialties and rheumatology is no exception. Cartilage repair is already possible, but relevant techniques are becoming increasingly sophisticated, and may ultimately provide therapies for osteoarthritis (page 83). Scientific advances also continue to enhance our understanding and treatment of a variety of rheumatic diseases, as exemplified by Sjögren's syndrome (page 57) and catastrophic antiphospholipid syndrome (page 89). Alongside these discoveries are parallel advances in our diagnostic capabilities. The introduction of ultrasound into rheumatology is set to revolutionize diagnosis and management of many conditions, including some types of vasculitis (page 67).

Fast Facts: Rheumatology Highlights 2005–06 brings together a diverse collection of topics written by internationally recognized experts. The opinions expressed in this handbook reflect those of the chapter authors, each of whom provides an interesting and stimulating update on recent advances in rheumatology.

John D Isaacs PhD FRCP
Professor of Clinical Rheumatology
University of Newcastle upon Tyne, UK

Current treatment of osteoarthritis

Peter Brooks MD FRACP FRCP Edin FAFRM FAFPHM
University of Queensland, Royal Brisbane Hospital, Australia

Nearly 10% of men and 20% of women aged 60 or more suffer from symptoms of osteoarthritis, and this number is increasing rapidly with the aging population.[1] This burgeoning epidemic of osteoarthritis was one of the major drivers for the creation of the Bone and Joint Decade (2000–2010), a global initiative intended to improve the lives of people with musculoskeletal disorders by advancing knowledge and treatment of these conditions through education and research.[2]

Osteoarthritis has been the 'poor cousin' of the inflammatory rheumatic diseases over the years, but times may be changing. Heightened interest in osteoarthritis research – such as the National Institutes of Health (NIH) Glucosamine/Chondroitin Arthritis Intervention Trial (GAIT) (see http://nccam.nih.gov/news/19972000/121100/qa.htm) and the osteoarthritis initiative, which is examining predictors of the condition (see www.niams.nih.gov/ne/oi/index.htm) – suggest that rheumatologists should now 'embrace osteoarthritis'.[3]

Management principles

Dieppe and Lohmander have carefully outlined the principles that must be reviewed when managing a patient with osteoarthritis (Figure 1).[4] They point out the challenge of focusing on patient needs and outcomes, and stress the importance of not overtreating or medicalizing patients with mild osteoarthritis, many of whom will cope very well with little or no medical intervention.

These authors also stress the need for individualized therapy with a combination of drug and non-drug treatments, reviewed at frequent intervals as the patient's symptoms and requirements change. Of significant concern in this regard is the need for more resources for joint replacement. Unfortunately, there are still

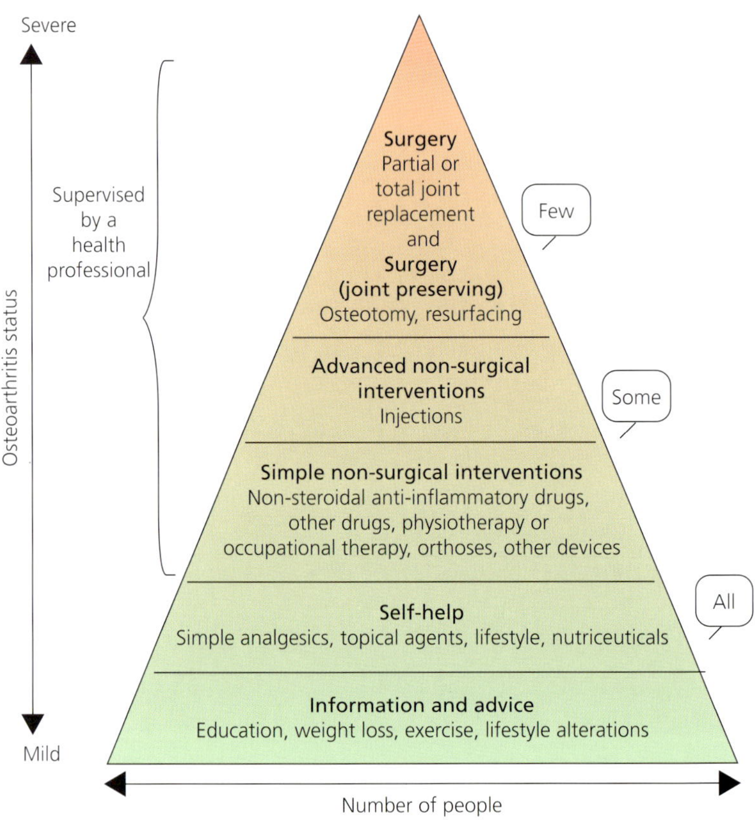

Figure 1 Principles for the management of osteoarthritis. Reproduced from Dieppe and Lohmander.[4] Copyright 2005, with permission of Elsevier.

significant barriers to patients with hip and knee pain and disability seeking adequate treatment – particularly in relation to surgery. There is little doubt that hip and knee replacements are some of the most cost-effective operations available, and most patients who have these operations do extraordinarily well. Pessimism about the availability of treatments, and concerns about effectiveness and the risks of surgery still make older people reluctant to seek medical help.[5] A treatment algorithm for the management of osteoarthritis of the hip and knee is shown in Figure 2,[6] and treatment options are discussed in the following sections.

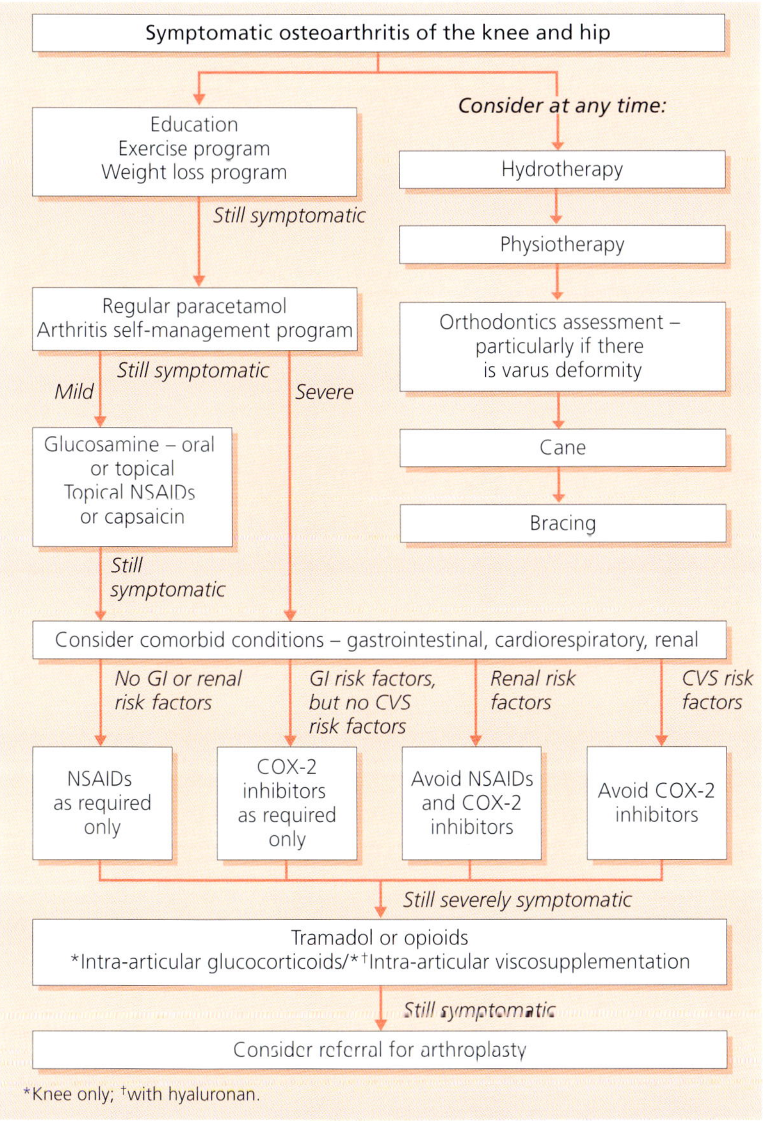

Figure 2 Management algorithm for osteoarthritis of the knee and hip. Reproduced from Grainger R and Cicuttini FM. Medical management of osteoarthritis of the knee and hip joints. *MJA* 2004;180:232–6, with permission of *The Medical Journal of Australia*. Copyright © 2004. COX-2, cyclooxygenase-2; CVS, cardiovascular system; GI, gastrointestinal; NSAIDs, non-steroidal anti-inflammatory drugs.

Exercise and physiotherapy programs

A trial comparing exercise therapy, monthly telephone contact, combined exercise therapy and telephone contact, and no intervention found that exercise therapy was more effective but associated with higher costs. While exercise therapy reduced knee pain, it did not lead to a reduction in the use of medical resources.[7] Compared with 'care as usual', a self-management program (six sessions of 2 hours each, led by physiotherapists) resulted in a significant reduction in pain and significant improvement in the Western Ontario and McMaster Universities (WOMAC) function score, which increased during a 21-month follow-up period.[8] Whilst these studies suggest benefit from exercise, a further study of physiotherapy that included exercises, massage, taping and mobilization was no different in outcome to a placebo regimen of sham ultrasound and light application of a non-therapeutic gel.[9]

Drug treatment

Non-steroidal anti-inflammatory drugs. The COX-1-sparing debate has once again focused concern (particularly of primary care providers and patients) on the use of all non-steroidal anti-inflammatory drugs (NSAIDs) for the management of osteoarthritis. It now seems clear that all NSAIDs are associated with a slight increase in the incidence of cardiovascular disease,[10] though this increase does seem to be somewhat greater with the potent COX-1-sparing agents.[11] What is clear from all research in this area is the significant underpowering of most studies to get a reasonable answer in terms of cardiovascular disease and NSAID use.

The principles of NSAID use for osteoarthritis are still as follows.

- Start with an adequate trial of non-pharmacological therapies and pure analgesics.
- If an NSAID is to be used, start with the mildest in terms of efficacy and side effects.
- Review treatment at frequent intervals to ensure the patient is not developing adverse events and is responding to therapy.

These principles are included by the Taskforce of the European League Against Rheumatism's (EULAR) Standing Committee for

International Clinical Studies Including Therapeutics (ESCISIT) in its report on the development of EULAR evidence-based guidelines for the management of hip osteoarthritis.[12] These guidelines can be readily adapted for other joints.

Recent reviews of topical NSAID use for chronic musculoskeletal pain continue to provide evidence of some efficacy with a low incidence of adverse events.[13]

Viscosupplementation. Although an internet-based, randomized controlled trial of glucosamine versus placebo failed to show differences between the patient groups at 12 weeks,[14] a major analysis of viscosupplementation for the treatment of osteoarthritis of the knee demonstrated efficacy with no major safety issues.[15] Interestingly, a meta-analysis of intra-articular corticosteroid treatment for osteoarthritis of the knee showed similar short-term benefit with few side effects, but little to support long-term efficacy.[16]

Doxycycline in the management of osteoarthritis has been the focus of interest for some years. In a recently reported 30-month study comparing doxycycline, 100 mg twice daily, with placebo, the rate of joint-space narrowing in knees with established osteoarthritis was slowed in the group receiving doxycycline. Interestingly, there was no effect on joint-space narrowing in the contralateral knee, suggesting that pathogenetic mechanisms in that joint are different from those in the index knee.[17]

Non-pharmacological management

Acupuncture is still used extensively for osteoarthritis. A recent study of acupuncture in the management of chronic osteoarthritis of the knee demonstrated that pain was significantly reduced and joint function was significantly improved with acupuncture compared with minimal or no acupuncture. However, these benefits decreased over time and were not sustained for 6 months.[18]

Patient education is of significant importance for individuals with osteoarthritis. Educational material must be made available.

Highlights in **current treatment of osteoarthritis** *2005–06*

WHAT'S IN?

- Use of evidence-based decisions for individual treatment plans
- Exercise and weight control
- Doxycycline (although cost–benefit studies are required)
- Total joint replacement

WHAT'S OUT?

- Non-steroidal anti-inflammatory drugs (NSAIDs), unless appropriate risk factors – both gastrointestinal and cardiovascular – are also addressed; if they are, NSAIDs (including COX-1-sparing agents) can be beneficial

WHAT'S NEEDED?

- Regular review of patients' therapeutic needs

References

1. Woolf AD, Pfleger B. Burden of major musculoskeletal conditions. *Bull World Health Organ* 2003;81: 646–56.

2. Hazes JM, Woolf AD. The bone and joint decade 2000–2010. *J Rheumatol* 2000;27:1–3.

3. Birrell F, Arden NK, Conaghan PG et al. Is it time for more rheumatologists to embrace osteoarthritis? *Rheumatology (Oxford)* 2005;44:829–30.

4. Dieppe PA, Lohmander LS. Pathogenesis and management of pain in osteoarthritis. *Lancet* 2005;365:965–73.

5. Sanders C, Donovan JL, Dieppe PA. Unmet need for joint replacement: a qualitative investigation of barriers to treatment among individuals with severe pain and disability of the hip and knee. *Rheumatology* 2004;43:353–7.

6. Grainger R, Cicuttini FM. Medical management of osteoarthritis of the knee and hip joints. *Med J Aust* 2004;180:232–6.

7. Thomas KS, Miller P, Doherty M et al. Cost-effectiveness of a two-year home exercise program for the treatment of knee pain. *Arthritis Rheum* 2005;53:388–94.

8. Heuts PH, de Bie R, Drietelaar M et al. Self-management in osteoarthritis of hip or knee: a randomized clinical trial in a primary healthcare setting. *J Rheumatol* 2005;32:543–9.

9. Bennell KL, Hinman RS, Metcalf BR et al. Efficacy of physiotherapy management of knee joint osteoarthritis: a randomised, double blind, placebo controlled trial. *Ann Rheum Dis* 2005;64:906–12.

10. Johnsen SP, Larsson H, Tarone RE et al. Risk of hospitalization for myocardial infarction among users of rofecoxib, celecoxib, and other NSAIDs: a population-based case-control study. *Arch Intern Med* 2005,165:978–84.

11. Ray WA, MacDonald TM, Solomon DH et al. COX-2 selective non-steroidal anti-inflammatory drugs and cardiovascular disease. *Pharmacoepidemiol Drug Saf* 2003;12:67–70.

12. Zhang W, Doherty M, Arden N et al. EULAR evidence based recommendations for the management of hip osteoarthritis: report of a task force of the EULAR Standing Committee for International Clinical Studies Including Therapeutics (ESCISIT). *Ann Rheum Dis* 2005;64:669–81.

13. Mason L, Moore RA, Edwards JE et al. Topical NSAIDs for chronic musculoskeletal pain: systematic review and meta-analysis. *BMC Musculoskelet Disord* 2004;5:28.

14. McAlindon T, Formica M, LaValley M et al. Effectiveness of glucosamine for symptoms of knee osteoarthritis: results from an internet-based randomized double-blind controlled trial. *Am J Med* 2004;117:643–9.

15. Bellamy N, Campbell J, Robinson V et al. Viscosupplementation for the treatment of osteoarthritis of the knee. *Cochrane Database Syst Rev* 2005; issue 2:CD005321. www.thecochranelibrary.com.

16. Bellamy N, Campbell J, Robinson V et al. Intraarticular corticosteroid for treatment of osteoarthritis of the knee. *Cochrane Database Syst Rev* 2005; issue 2:CD005328. www.thecochranelibrary.com.

17. Brandt KD, Mazzuca SA, Katz BP et al. Effects of doxycycline on progression of osteoarthritis: results of a randomized, placebo-controlled, double-blind trial. *Arthritis Rheum* 2005;52:2015–25.

18. Witt C, Brinkhaus B, Jena S et al. Acupuncture in patients with osteoarthritis of the knee: a randomised trial. *Lancet* 2005; 366:136–43.

Risks and benefits of COX-2 inhibitors

Vibeke Strand* MD and Lee S Simon† MD
*Division of Immunology, Stanford University, California, USA
†Harvard Medical School, Beth Israel Deaconess Center, Massachusetts, USA

Non-selective non-steroidal anti-inflammatory drugs (NS-NSAIDs) and cyclooxygenase-2 selective agents (COX-2 inhibitors) have, despite the controversies surrounding their use, been proven equally effective in the treatment of acute and chronic pain and of inflammatory arthritis. As our population ages, the use of these drugs will necessarily increase, requiring us to better decipher their similarities and differences.

Gastrointestinal safety

Although the 'large, simple trials' – Vioxx Gastrointestinal Outcomes Research (VIGOR), the Celecoxib Long-term Arthritis Safety Study (CLASS) and, subsequently, the Therapeutic Arthritis Research and Gastrointestinal Event Trial (TARGET) – differed in conduct, comparator arms and outcome measures, it is clear that the COX-2 inhibitors conferred a better gastrointestinal (GI) safety profile than the NS-NSAIDs.

If the same combined endpoint of documented GI ulcers and their complications (i.e. perforations, obstruction and bleeds) is applied to all available data across all three randomized controlled trials (RCTs), rofecoxib, celecoxib and lumiracoxib are associated with fewer events than are naproxen, diclofenac and ibuprofen.

Risk of thromboembolic cardiovascular events

'Prevention' trials. An increased risk of thromboembolic cardiovascular (CV) events associated with the administration of rofecoxib was first reported in VIGOR. Subsequently, placebo controlled trials designed to demonstrate the benefits of COX-2 inhibitors in the prevention of colonic polyps (Adenomatous Polyp

Prevention On Vioxx [APPROVe], Adenoma Prevention with Celecoxib [APC] and Prevention of Spontaneous Adenomatous Polyposis [PreSAP] trials) and the prevention of Alzheimer's disease (Alzheimer's Disease Anti-inflammatory Prevention Trial [ADAPT]), identified an increased risk of CV events with celecoxib and the NS-NSAID naproxen sodium, as well as with rofecoxib.[1–4]

All four trials were stopped early because of ethical considerations; only published data from APPROVe allowed the recurrence of polyps to be compared with the incidence of thromboembolic CV events. Colonoscopy data from the other two RCTs are not yet available and detailed information from the ADAPT RCT is still eagerly awaited. Thus, it is not possible to weigh the potential risks against the potential benefits in these populations. This is disappointing, as these studies represent the few long-term protocols to have included a placebo treatment arm.

It is important to be aware that thromboembolic CV events were not predefined endpoints in any of the 'prevention' RCTs – analyses were retrospectively applied when epidemiological studies, following the VIGOR findings, continued to indicate a potentially increased risk of CV events associated with the COX-2 inhibitors, particularly rofecoxib. Discontinuing a trial before the estimated accrual and treatment exposure are completed exposes results to unanticipated effects of treating and reporting bias. Such studies may not reveal true treatment differences unless, as in VIGOR and APPROVe, a 'signal' continues to manifest over time once it has been identified.

Further data on cardiovascular risk. Subsequent to the findings of VIGOR, epidemiological studies repeatedly demonstrated an increased risk of acute myocardial infarction (MI), hypertension and congestive heart failure (CHF) with rofecoxib at doses above 25 mg/day compared with celecoxib and NS-NSAIDs.[5–7]

The results of a large 1.4-million cohort study from Kaiser Permanente, published in 2005, revealed statistically increased risks for acute MI and sudden death with NS-NSAIDs, specifically indometacin, naproxen and 'other NSAIDs' (approaching significance with diclofenac and ibuprofen), as well as with rofecoxib (> 25 mg/day).[8]

Data from the largest inception cohort study of acute MI in 1.9 million patients in the California Medi-Cal database have also been reported recently.[9] Administration of rofecoxib above 25 mg/day was associated with a definite increased risk of acute MI, while lower doses were associated with a probable increased risk. There was evidence that the increased risk began early, within the first 30 days of use, consistent with previously published data from Ray and Solomon.[10,11] A probable increased risk was evident with celecoxib doses above 200 mg/day, but there was no apparent risk with valdecoxib at doses of 10–20 mg/day. Statistically significant increased risks were associated with indometacin, sulindac, ibuprofen and meloxicam; naproxen did not confer cardioprotection.

Other published results have demonstrated an increased risk of CV events associated with the use of NS-NSAIDs, and have confirmed differences between rofecoxib and celecoxib. In the UK General Practice Database, the risk of acute MI increased within 3 months of prescribing rofecoxib, ibuprofen, diclofenac and naproxen, but not celecoxib.[12]

In a combined North American insurance claims database of patients with rheumatoid arthritis, use of naproxen and rofecoxib was associated with an increased risk of hospitalization for CHF, compared with a decreased risk with celecoxib or any disease-modifying antirheumatic drug.[13]

In Quebec, the risk of recurrent CHF or death was significantly lower in those prescribed celecoxib than in those who took NS-NSAIDs or rofecoxib.[14]

In a small, nested case-control study in heavy smokers in Norway, researchers showed that long-term use of NS-NSAIDs reduced the risk of oral cancer by approximately 50%, yet did not result in survival differences over 5–29 years because of a statistically increased risk of CV-related death.[15]

Explaining the data

The data with NS-NSAIDs further confound the 'imbalance hypothesis' that selective COX-2 inhibition without concomitant inhibition of COX-1 activity may result in an increased risk of thrombosis.

Destabilization of blood pressure. Other explanations, possibly more evidence based, include the renal effects of COX-2 inhibition. Although COX-2 production is largely inducible by inflammatory stimuli, COX-2 is constitutively produced in the kidney and brain and during ovulation. Inhibition of COX-2 activity in the macula densa of the proximal tubule leads to salt and water retention, resulting in similar increases in blood pressure and edema as observed with NS-NSAID treatment, albeit through a different mechanism. Across RCTs, increases in blood pressure and peripheral edema were observed with COX-2 inhibitors as well as with comparator NS-NSAIDs; the increases were higher with rofecoxib, which showed a dose–response effect at 12.5, 25 and 50 mg/day.

A meta-analysis by Aw et al. of RCT data published before May 2004 confirmed a differential effect for the development of hypertension with rofecoxib compared with celecoxib.[16]

A prospective trial in approximately 400 patients with osteoarthritis, hypertension (treated with angiotensin-converting-enzyme [ACE] inhibitors) and diabetes compared 24-hour ambulatory blood pressure measurements in patients receiving rofecoxib, celecoxib and naproxen.[17] Although blood pressure control was destabilized in all groups, destabilization was more frequent with rofecoxib treatment, which resulted in statistically significant increases in systolic blood pressure of 3–4 mmHg above that reported with naproxen and celecoxib throughout the 24-hour period at 6 weeks.

Messerli and Sichrovsky argue convincingly that these small increases in systolic blood pressure are sufficient to explain the excess of CV events observed with rofecoxib in APPROVe, with high-dose celecoxib treatment in APC and with naproxen in ADAPT.[18] Importantly, the number of cerebrovascular accidents, as well as MIs, increased in APPROVe, and aspirin did not confer protection against these events, suggesting underlying blood pressure destabilization. Thus, all patients receiving NS-NSAIDs or COX-2 inhibitors should be carefully monitored and treated aggressively for changes in blood pressure.

Mechanistic differences. Are there mechanistic hypotheses that could explain the differential effects on blood pressure and edema – and the relative differences in the risk of CV events – between the COX-2 inhibitors? It is clear that rofecoxib and celecoxib differ in structure, COX-2 selectivity, plasma-protein binding, pharmacokinetics and metabolism.[19] A metabolite of rofecoxib may inhibit the metabolism of aldosterone, and celecoxib may exhibit carbonic anhydrase activity.

Hermann et al. compared rofecoxib, celecoxib, diclofenac and placebo in Dahl rats with salt-sensitive hypertension.[20] Celecoxib administration decreased proteinuria and histological evidence of glomerular and vascular injury when compared with the effects of diclofenac and rofecoxib. Rofecoxib dramatically worsened proteinuria and glomerular inflammation and increased the endothelial dysfunction associated with lower endothelial nitric oxide synthase mRNA. These observations confirm previous data in the same model, which showed that celecoxib reduced endothelial dysfunction and oxidative stress, while rofecoxib and diclofenac exerted no effect.

Clinical studies in patients with coronary artery disease or hypertension have also shown that celecoxib improves vascular endothelial function. Together, these data implicate oxidative stress as a potential mechanism underlying some of the deleterious effects observed with rofecoxib.

The US position

Amid the controversies, a Food and Drug Administration (FDA) Advisory Panel was convened in the hope that a public hearing, open to all interested parties (and available by videotape and videocast, and broadcast on US television), would help to clarify the issues.[4]

Highlights in **risks and benefits of COX-2 inhibitors** *2005–06*

WHAT'S IN?

- Continued use of COX-2 selective agents:
  - in patients with chronic pain, with high risk of gastrointestinal (GI) complications
  - for pre-emptive anesthesia
- Recognition that even a 2–3 mmHg increase in systolic blood pressure and/or diastolic blood pressure may increase the risk of thromboembolic cardiovascular (CV) events with *any* COX-2 inhibitor or non-selective non-steroidal anti-inflammatory drug (NS-NSAID)
- Awareness that, as with NS-NSAIDs, not all COX-2 inhibitors are alike – individual responses differ

WHAT'S OUT?

- The 'COX imbalance' hypothesis
- Widespread use of NS-NSAIDs or COX-2 inhibitors in everyone with chronic pain, without consideration of:
  - underlying GI risk factors
  - underlying CV risk factors, including hypertension and congestive heart failure
  - use of low-dose prophylactic aspirin

WHAT'S NEEDED?

- Definitive evaluation of CV risk with celecoxib, valdecoxib/parecoxib, etoricoxib, lumiracoxib and NS-NSAIDs, including naproxen
- Thoughtful, evidence-based recommendations

During the debate that followed, the view of non-clinical epidemiologists, safety experts and statisticians 'trumped' the opinion of clinical rheumatologists, cardiologists, nephrologists, anesthesiologists, neurologists, psychologists and general internists – all treating physicians. Despite the votes taken at this meeting, which concluded that the available data supported marketing of all three COX-2 inhibitors in the USA, only one remains available. In our opinion, this is unfortunate as, like NS-NSAIDs, COX-2 inhibitors behave differently in different individuals, and not all patients respond to a single agent within a class. Every practicing physician should be able to weigh the potential benefits for an individual patient against the potential risks of a prescribed therapy, particularly those designed for chronic use.

In June 2005, the FDA published its requirement that all NS-NSAIDs (including over-the-counter ibuprofen and naproxen sodium) and COX-2 inhibitors should carry a 'black box warning' to highlight the potential increased risk of CV events and life-threatening GI-bleeding events. This action further underscores the importance of considering the potential increased risk of CV events associated with the use of any and all of the anti-inflammatory agents.

A final note

In view of the continuing controversies, the evidence-based recommendations proposed by the Canadian Consensus are particularly welcome.[21]

References

1. Bresalier RS, Sandler RS, Quan H et al.; Adenomatous Polyp Prevention on Vioxx (APPROVe) Trial Investigators. Cardiovascular events associated with rofecoxib in a colorectal adenoma chemoprevention trial. *N Engl J Med* 2005;352: 1092–102.

2. Solomon SD, McMurray JJ, Pfeffer MA et al.; Adenoma Prevention with Celecoxib (APC) Study Investigators. Cardiovascular risk associated with celecoxib in a clinical trial for colorectal adenoma prevention. *N Engl J Med* 2005; 352:1071–80.

3. FDA Advisory Committee Briefing Document. Celecoxib and Valdecoxib Cardiovascular Safety. January 12, 2005. www.fda.gov/ohrms/dockets/ac/05/briefing/2005-4090B1_03_Pfizer-Celebrex-Bextra.pdf

4. Summary minutes from the Joint Meeting of the FDA Arthritis Advisory Committee and the Drug Safety and Risk Management Advisory Committee. February 16–18, 2005, Gaithersburg, Maryland, USA. www.fda.gov/ohrms/dockets/ac/05/minutes/2005-4090M1_Final.htm

5. Johnsen SP, Larsson H, Tarone RE et al. Risk of hospitalization for myocardial infarction among users of rofecoxib, celecoxib, and other NSAIDS: a population-based case-control study. *Arch Intern Med* 2005;165:978–84.

6. Kimmel SE, Berlin JA, Reilly M et al. Patients exposed to rofecoxib and celecoxib have different odds of nonfatal myocardial infarction. *Ann Intern Med* 2005;142:157–64.

7. Levesque LE, Brophy JM, Zhang B. The risk of myocardial infarction with cyclooxygenase-2 inhibitors: a population study of elderly adults. *Ann Intern Med* 2005;142:481–9.

8. Graham DJ, Campen D, Hui R et al. Risk of acute myocardial infarction and sudden cardiac death in patients treated with cyclo-oxygenase 2 selective and non-selective non-steroidal anti-inflammatory drugs: nested case-control study. *Lancet* 2005;365:475–81.

9. Singh G, Mithal A, Triadafilopoulos G. Both selective COX-2 inhibitors and non-selective NSAIDs increase the risk of acute myocardial infarction in patients with arthritis: selectivity is with the patient, not the drug class. *Ann Rheum Dis* 2005;64(suppl III):85 [abstr.].

10. Ray WA, Stein CM, Hall K et al. Non-steroidal anti-inflammatory drugs and risk of serious coronary heart disease: an observational cohort study. *Lancet* 2002;359:118–23.

11. Solomon DH, Schneeweiss S, Glynn RJ et al. Relationship between selective cyclooxygenase-2 inhibitors and acute myocardial infarction in older adults. *Circulation* 2004;109:2068–73.

12. Hippisley-Cox J, Coupland C. Risk of myocardial infarction in patients taking cyclo-oxygenase-2 inhibitors or conventional non-steroidal anti-inflammatory drugs: population based nested case-control analysis. *BMJ* 2005;330:1366–72.

13. Bernatsky S, Hudson M, Suissa S. Anti-rheumatic drug use and risk of hospitalization for congestive heart failure in rheumatoid arthritis. *Rheumatology (Oxford)* 2005;44:677–80.

14. Hudson M, Richard H, Pilote L. Differences in outcomes of patients with congestive heart failure prescribed celecoxib, rofecoxib, or non-steroidal anti-inflammatory drugs: population based study. *BMJ* 2005;330:1370–5.

15. Sudbo J, Lee JJ, Lippman SM et al. Non-steroidal anti-inflammatory drugs and the risk of oral cancer: a nested case-control study. *Lancet* 2005;366:1359–66.

16. Aw TJ, Hass SJ, Liew D, Krum H. Meta-analysis of cyclooxygenase-2 inhibitors and their effects on blood pressure. *Arch Intern Med* 2005; 165:490–6.

17. Sowers, JR, White WB, Pitt B et al.; Celecoxib Rofecoxib Efficacy and Safety in Comorbidities Evaluation Trial (CRESCENT) Investigators. The effects of cyclooxygenase-2 inhibitors and nonsteroidal anti-inflammatory therapy on 24-hour blood pressure in patients with hypertension, osteoarthritis and type 2 diabetes mellitus. *Arch Intern Med* 2005;165: 161–8; erratum 2005;165:551.

18. Messerli FH, Sichrovsky T. Does the pro-hypertensive effect of cyclooxygenase-2 inhibitors account for the increased risk in cardiovascular disease? *Am J Cardiol* 2005;96:872–3.

19. Chang IJ, Harris RC. Are all COX-2 inhibitors created equal? *Hypertension* 2005;45:178–80.

20. Hermann M, Shaw S, Kiss E et al. Selective COX-2 inhibitors and renal injury in salt-sensitive hypertension. *Hypertension* 2005;45:193–7.

21. Tannenbaum H, Bombardier C, Davis P et al. An evidence-based approach to prescribing nonsteroidal antiinflammatory drugs. Third Canadian Consensus Conference. *J Rheumatol* 2006;33:140–57.

When does rheumatoid arthritis begin?

Dirkjan van Schaardenburg[*†] MD PhD,
Irene van der Horst-Bruinsma[†] MD PhD and Ben Dijkmans[*†] MD PhD
Departments of Rheumatology, *Jan van Breemen Institute, Amsterdam
†VU University Medical Center, Amsterdam, The Netherlands

When does rheumatoid arthritis (RA) begin? It's a seemingly straightforward question that has the potential to cause much academic debate. In a simple disease such as influenza, the beginning can be assumed to occur shortly after the first contact with the offending virus. Atherosclerotic vascular disease, as a different example, mostly has a long asymptomatic phase of plaque formation without any signs or symptoms. If, during that period, an aortic aneurysm is found unexpectedly on abdominal sonography, performed for some other reason, most physicians will agree that a disease is present. If one looks for it, one will find a lot of subclinical or preclinical vascular disease in the form of atherosclerotic plaques.

'False-positive' rheumatoid factor

Now let us focus on RA. This disease is thought to be caused by the interplay of partly known genetic and environmental factors, and at some point in time symptomatic arthritis occurs. Until a decade ago, nobody was in much of a hurry to treat RA, as the course of the disease did not seem to be significantly modified by the available interventions. At that time it was obvious when the disease actually started, that is, when the arthritis started. Until recently, many rheumatologists would consider that a patient with joint pain but no joint swelling and with a positive rheumatoid factor (RF) was not at high risk for RA. The RF positivity would be considered to be a 'false positive' because RF is not very specific for RA.

Early diagnosis and treatment

After it became clear that RA could be treated effectively, there was an increasing drive to treat the disease early in order to avoid joint damage. However, as the treatment is potentially toxic, we must identify who really needs it – in other words, to find the individuals with 'real' RA. In recognizing potentially disabling early disease, the classic American College of Rheumatology (ACR) criteria for RA proved to be problematic. This does not come as a surprise as these criteria were developed to distinguish between different forms of established arthritis.

Therefore, in early polyarthritis, interest has shifted away from the formal diagnosis of RA towards prognostic features to guide treatment decisions. Recently developed tests for antibodies against citrullinated proteins (ACPA) or against cyclic citrullinated peptides (anti-CCP), which are highly specific for RA, have proven very helpful in this respect. Several authors have found that the presence of anti-CCP antibodies predicts more severe disease.[1,2] Another argument for the importance of these antibodies is the finding of a functional link between RA-specific human leukocyte antigen (HLA) haplotypes (in particular, *HLA-DR4*) and the production of ACPA.[3]

These antibodies (Table 1) may help to identify patients with developing RA who need treatment but who do not yet satisfy the ACR criteria. Indeed, a recent paper identifies anti-CCP as an

TABLE 1

Properties of antibodies against citrullinated proteins

- Present before symptoms emerge in half of patients
- More sensitive and specific for RA than RF
- Only partially overlap with RF
- Associated with *HLA-DR4*-positive RA
- Locally produced in inflamed joints
- Predict a worse outcome in RA

HLA, human leukocyte antigen; RA, rheumatoid arthritis; RF, rheumatoid factor.

accurate predictor of the development of undifferentiated arthritis into RA.[4] This may have consequences for the treatment of early arthritis. A trial completed in 2005 showed that the progression of undifferentiated arthritis to RA can be diminished by methotrexate treatment.[5] Other trials are under way that apply potent antirheumatic drugs in patients with oligoarthritis.

Arthralgia or arthritis?

Established RA is easily recognized, and most physicians will agree that the same disease – RA – is present in the early phase of arthritis (i.e. before the ACR criteria are satisfied). The situation becomes less clear cut if persistent arthritis is preceded by a phase of joint pain. If this phase is accompanied by intermittent joint swelling, a diagnosis of palindromic rheumatism is often applied. A substantial proportion of these patients will develop RA in time: in particular, those with a positive test for RF and probably those with anti-CCP positivity.[6] However, there are no data on the risk of developing RA for a person with arthralgia with or without RA-specific autoantibodies.

Moreover, it has become necessary to further define what is meant by 'arthritis'. Ultrasonography and magnetic resonance imaging studies have shown evidence of synovitis that was not apparent on clinical examination. In patients with oligoarthritis, ultrasonography revealed synovitis in 33% of painful non-swollen joints and in 13% of painless non-swollen joints.[7] Although the clinical significance of 'imaging synovitis' is yet to be established, it seems that the detection of synovitis by physical examination – apart from having suboptimal reproducibility – has low sensitivity.

Preclinical rheumatoid arthritis

Fifteen years ago, antikeratin antibodies (a type of ACPA) were demonstrated in people who developed RA years later. Two recent studies show the development of anti-CCP antibodies and RF in serial blood samples from donors in the years before RA symptoms started.[8,9] In half of the patients, an elevated RF was found at a median of 2 years and an elevated anti-CCP was found at a median

Highlights in when does rheumatoid arthritis begin? *2005–06*

WHAT'S IN?

- Testing for antibodies to citrullinated proteins
- Ultrasonography for suspected arthritis
- Recognition that smoking is a risk factor for (more severe) rheumatoid arthritis (RA)

WHAT'S OUT?

- Using American College of Rheumatology criteria to diagnose early RA
- Postponing disease-modifying antirheumatic drug treatment in early RA

WHAT'S NEEDED?

- Prospective studies that tell us whether treatment of antibody-positive asymptomatic individuals reduces progression to RA

of 5 years before symptoms emerged.[9] This immunologic derangement is accompanied by systemic inflammation, as measured by C-reactive protein and soluble phospholipase A2, which is only slightly less in those without autoantibodies.[10,11] Alterations in markers of osteoclast activation are present before the start of symptoms and are even predictive of the later degree of bone destruction.[12] Therefore, several parameters that are indicative of RA are already abnormal in the years before symptoms emerge in many patients. The next step will be to look for the presence of histological synovitis in these people, as has been demonstrated in joints not yet clinically affected in patients with RA.[13]

In this phase, environmental factors may affect the risk of developing arthritis. An example of a risk enhancer is smoking.[14] A high consumption of antioxidants is a risk reducer.[15] Overall, the risk of developing RA within 5 years in asymptomatic people with anti-CCP is 5%, which increases to 69% in multicase families.[9]

Conclusion

The fact that immunologic and biochemical alterations typical of RA occur many years before the symptoms emerge has shifted the answer to the question 'when does RA begin?' well into a phase in which people still feel healthy.

The recent term 'preclinical RA' is used to define people with antibodies but not arthritis. This is a very interesting group of people in which to study the pathogenesis of RA, but to them the only relevant – and, for the time being, unanswered – question is whether an intervention will become available that has advantages over the current approach to treat only symptomatic (poly)arthritis.

A double-blind randomized trial of two dexamethasone injections versus placebo is now in progress in the hope of substantially lowering antibody concentrations in the short term and of reducing progression to RA in the long term in these people.

References

1. Visser H, le Cessie S, Vos K et al. How to diagnose rheumatoid arthritis early: a prediction model for persistent (erosive) arthritis. *Arthritis Rheum* 2002;46:357–65.

2. Nielen MM, van der Horst AR, van Schaardenburg D et al. Antibodies to citrullinated human fibrinogen (ACF) have diagnostic and prognostic value in early arthritis. *Ann Rheum Dis* 2005;64: 1199–204.

3. Berglin E, Padyukov L, Sundin U et al. A combination of autoantibodies to cyclic citrullinated peptide (CCP) and HLA-DRB1 locus antigens is strongly associated with future onset of rheumatoid arthritis. *Arthritis Res Ther* 2004;6:R303–8.

4. van Gaalen FA, Linn-Rasker SP, van Venrooij WJ et al. Autoantibodies to cyclic citrullinated peptides predict progression to rheumatoid arthritis in patients with undifferentiated arthritis: a prospective cohort study. *Arthritis Rheum* 2004;50:709–15.

5. van Dongen H, van Aken J, Lard LR et al. Treatment of patients with undifferentiated arthritis with methotrexate: a double-blind placebo-controlled randomized clinical trial. *Arthritis Rheum* 2005;51S:L4/479.

6. Salvador G, Gomez A, Vinas O et al. Prevalence and clinical significance of anti-cyclic citrullinated peptide and antikeratin antibodies in palindromic rheumatism. An abortive form of rheumatoid arthritis? *Rheumatology (Oxford)* 2003;42:972–5.

7. Wakefield RJ, Green MJ, Marzo-Ortega H et al. Should oligoarthritis be reclassified? Ultrasound reveals a high prevalence of subclinical disease. *Ann Rheum Dis* 2004;63:382–5.

8. Rantapaa-Dahlqvist S, de Jong BA, Berglin E et al. Antibodies against cyclic citrullinated peptide and IgA rheumatoid factor predict the development of rheumatoid arthritis. *Arthritis Rheum* 2003;48:2741–9.

9. Nielen MM, van Schaardenburg D, Reesink HW et al. Specific autoantibodies precede the symptoms of rheumatoid arthritis: a study of serial measurements in blood donors. *Arthritis Rheum* 2004;50:380–6.

10. Nielen MM, van Schaardenburg D, Reesink HW et al. Increased levels of C-reactive protein in serum from blood donors before the onset of rheumatoid arthritis. *Arthritis Rheum* 2004;50:2423–7.

11. Nielen MM, van Schaardenburg D, Reesink HW et al. Simultaneous development of acute phase response and autoantibodies in preclinical rheumatoid arthritis. *Ann Rheum Dis* 2005; Aug 3 [Epub ahead of print].

12. Nielen MM, van Schaardenburg D, Twisk JWR et al. Markers of bone formation and resorption in preclinical rheumatoid arthritis are associated with radiographic progression. *Arthritis Rheum* 2005;51S:1538.

13. Kraan MC, Versendaal H, Jonker M et al. Asymptomatic synovitis precedes clinically manifest arthritis. *Arthritis Rheum* 1998;41:1481–8.

14. Padyukov L, Silva C, Stolt P et al. A gene–environment interaction between smoking and shared epitope genes in HLA-DR provides a high risk of seropositive rheumatoid arthritis. *Arthritis Rheum* 2004;50:3085–92.

15. Pattison DJ, Symmons DP, Lunt M et al. Dietary beta-cryptoxanthin and inflammatory polyarthritis: results from a population-based prospective study. *Am J Clin Nutr* 2005;82:451–5.

Genetics of rheumatoid arthritis

Jane Worthington PhD

ARC Epidemiology Research Unit, University of Manchester, UK

While it has long been established that susceptibility to rheumatoid arthritis (RA) is influenced by a combination of multiple genetic and environmental factors, since the identification of human leukocyte antigen (HLA)-*DRB1* as the major genetic factor approximately 30 years ago, progress towards identifying non-HLA genetic susceptibility or severity factors has been disappointing. In common with many other complex diseases, a number of linkage studies in affected sibling pair families have been carried out. However, based on our current understanding of the likely effect sizes of the genes we seek (odds ratio [OR] as low as 1.1–1.4), these have been underpowered.

There have also been hundreds, if not thousands, of genetic associations claimed for RA, but the common theme has been one of failure to replicate between studies, even within the same populations. This can be accounted for mainly by poor study design, in particular inadequate sample sizes, poor matching of cases and controls, insufficient or inappropriate markers and poor-quality genotyping.

This review is, however, timely in that, as a result of the dramatic advances in genetics over the last few years (completion of the genome sequence, identification of millions of single nucleotide polymorphisms [SNPs] and the characterization of these markers in different populations through the HapMap project) and the huge technological advances in genotyping methodologies (which have reduced the cost of high-throughput, high-quality genotyping), a second RA susceptibility gene *PTPN22* (encoding protein tyrosine phosphatase PTPN22, also known as Lyp) has been identified. In addition, since the initial report, identification of this gene has been replicated in every one of the ten studies that have followed.

Encouragingly, a number of other RA candidate genes emerged in 2005 from well-designed studies that have combined the developments listed above with investigation of the functional significance of the associated polymorphisms. While none of these has yet achieved the level of consensus seen for *PTPN22*, the future for RA genetics finally looks far more encouraging.

Protein tyrosine phosphatase N22 (*PTPN22*)

Lyp is a negative regulator of T-cell activation, and was targeted for investigation by researchers working on type 1 diabetes who found an association with a missense SNP (1858C→T).[1] Functional studies demonstrated that the disease-associated W620 variant reduced binding to Csk, the intracellular kinase that activates Lyp. It was hypothesized that carriage of the risk allele results in T cells with less effective downregulation and individuals who may, therefore, have an increased risk of developing an autoimmune response, although recent data suggest that the risk allele is in fact a gain-of-function variant.[2]

Association with rheumatoid arthritis. At the same time as the diabetes report, a large-scale study of 16 000 SNPs in candidate genes for RA found the strongest association (in a test cohort of 475 cases and controls) with exactly the same SNP in *PTPN22* as was identified in the diabetes study. In this elegant study, Begovich et al. replicated their results in a larger cohort of 840 cases and 840 controls (OR 2.1, $p = 3.4 \times 10^{-9}$) and demonstrated the functional effect of the polymorphism on binding to Csk.[3]

What then followed is unprecedented in the RA literature. Studies from the UK,[4,5] Spain,[6] Norway,[7] the Netherlands,[8] Canada,[9] New Zealand[10] and Finland[11] confirmed the association of the 1858C→T SNP with RA. Indeed, there appears to be only one contentious issue across all these studies and that is with respect to rheumatoid factor. Some studies did not detect the association in seronegative patients. However, in most of the studies the majority of patients were seropositive, and thus even the larger series may have been underpowered to detect an effect in the seronegative subgroups.

The most recent investigation of RA and *PTPN22* is the first to explore polymorphisms other than the 1858C→T SNP, and reports additional independent associations within the gene.[12] This may mean that *PTPN22* is even more important for RA susceptibility than first appeared to be the case. This observation must be followed up in those autoimmune diseases with no evidence of an association with the 1858C→T SNP.

In other diseases. It should also be noted that the importance of *PTPN22* is not restricted to RA and type 1 diabetes. This polymorphism has been investigated in other rheumatic and autoimmune diseases. Associations with systemic lupus erythematosus,[13,14] and most subgroups of juvenile idiopathic arthritis,[4] but not with systemic sclerosis or psoriatic arthritis,[4] have been reported. Other autoimmune diseases found to be associated with *PTPN22* include Hashimoto's thyroiditis,[15] Graves' disease[16–18] and Addison's disease.[17]

Peptidylarginine deiminase-4 (*PADI4*)

PADI4 first emerged as a candidate gene in 2003 from a Japanese study carrying out whole-genome-screening association studies.[19] As the enzyme responsible for post-translational citrullination of proteins (the target of anti-citrullinated peptide antibodies found in the sera of RA patients – see page 25), *PADI4* makes an attractive candidate gene for RA. The associated 4-SNP haplotype was found to result in greater mRNA stability.

In 2005, a convincing replication was reported in an independent Japanese cohort.[20] However, attempts at replication in other populations have been disappointing, with many negative studies.[21,22] A submission to the 2005 American College of Rheumatology annual general meeting described an association study of 25 SNPs in *PADI4* in a US cohort of patients with RA. A weak association with one of the SNPs on the Japanese haplotype and a strong association with an SNP in strong linkage disequilibrium (LD) provide the first evidence of association of *PADI4* in a non-Asian RA population.[23]

Highlights in **genetics of rheumatoid arthritis** *2005–06*

WHAT'S IN?

- Discovery of *PTPN22* – a genuine rheumatoid arthritis susceptibility gene
- Association studies based on well-designed and appropriately powered research
- Functional validation of associated polymorphisms
- Replication and validation in independent disease cohorts and different populations

WHAT'S OUT?

- Claims of genetic associations based on underpowered, poorly designed studies

Other potential susceptibility genes

Using a filter to select only the positive associations emerging from well-designed studies – that is, those with large sample sizes of well-characterized cases, presenting, when possible, evidence of independent replication or functional validation of associated polymorphisms – three further genes should be noted. In each case, however, more evidence of replication will be required before they can be considered alongside *PTPN22*. They are:

- the Fc-receptor-like gene (*FCRL3*),[24]
- the solute carrier family 22 gene (*SLC22A4*)[25]
- the MHC class II transactivator gene (*MHC2TA*).[26]

Associations with SNPs in the first two of these were identified in Japanese studies, but again have yet to be confirmed in non Asian populations, perhaps emphasizing the importance of genetic heterogeneity in RA.

The future

We can now be confident that as researchers exploit the enormous amount of data available on genetic polymorphisms to study large, well-characterized RA cohorts, more non-HLA susceptibility genes will be identified. It is worth bearing in mind that the transition from 'potential' to 'definite' disease gene ultimately requires a substantial body of genetic evidence and basic biology, as is so aptly illustrated by the *PTPN22* story that has unfolded during the past year.

References

1. Bottini N, Musumeci L, Alonso A et al. A functional variant of lymphoid tyrosine phosphatase is associated with type I diabetes. *Nat Genet* 2004;36:337–8.

2. Vang T, Congia M, Macis MD et al. Autoimmune-associated lymphoid tyrosine phosphatase is a gain-of-function variant. *Nat Genet* 2005;37:1317–19.

3. Begovich AB, Carlton VE, Honigberg LA et al. A missense single-nucleotide polymorphism in a gene encoding a protein tyrosine phosphatase (PTPN22) is associated with rheumatoid arthritis. *Am J Hum Genet* 2004;75:330–7.

4. Hinks A, Barton A, John S et al. Association between the PTPN22 gene and rheumatoid arthritis and juvenile idiopathic arthritis in a UK population: further support that PTPN22 is an autoimmunity gene. *Arthritis Rheum* 2005;52:1694–9.

5. Steer S, Lad B, Grumley JA et al. Association of R602W in a protein tyrosine phosphatase gene with a high risk of rheumatoid arthritis in a British population: evidence for an early onset/disease severity effect. *Arthritis Rheum* 2005;52:358–60.

6. Orozco G, Sanchez E, Gonzalez-Gay MA et al. Association of a functional single-nucleotide polymorphism of PTPN22, encoding lymphoid protein phosphatase, with rheumatoid arthritis and systemic lupus erythematosus. *Arthritis Rheum* 2005;52:219–24.

7. Viken MK, Amundsen SS, Kvien TK et al. Association analysis of the 1858C>T polymorphism in the PTPN22 gene in juvenile idiopathic arthritis and other autoimmune diseases. *Genes Immun* 2005;6: 271–3.

8. Zhernakova A, Eerligh P, Wijmenga C et al. Differential association of the PTPN22 coding variant with autoimmune diseases in a Dutch population. *Genes Immun* 2005;6:459–61.

9. van Oene M, Wintle RF, Liu X et al. Association of the lymphoid tyrosine phosphatase R620W variant with rheumatoid arthritis, but not Crohn's disease, in Canadian populations. *Arthritis Rheum* 2005;52:1993–8.

10. Simkins HM, Merriman ME, Highton J et al. Association of the PTPN22 locus with rheumatoid arthritis in a New Zealand Caucasian cohort. *Arthritis Rheum* 2005;52: 2222–5.

11. Seldin MF, Shigeta R, Laiho K et al. Finnish case-control and family studies support PTPN22 R620W polymorphism as a risk factor in rheumatoid arthritis, but suggest only minimal or no effect in juvenile idiopathic arthritis. *Genes Immun* 2005;6:720–2.

12. Carlton VE, Hu X, Chokkalingam AP et al. PTPN22 genetic variation: evidence for multiple variants associated with rheumatoid arthritis. *Am J Hum Genet* 2005;77:567–81.

13. Kyogoku C, Langefeld CD, Ortmann WA et al. Genetic association of the R620W polymorphism of protein tyrosine phosphatase PTPN22 with human SLE. *Am J Hum Genet* 2004;75:504–7.

14. Reddy MV, Johansson M, Sturfelt G et al. The R620W C/T polymorphism of the gene PTPN22 is associated with SLE independently of the association of PDCD1. *Genes Immun* 2005;6:658–62.

15. Criswell LA, Pfeiffer KA, Lum RF et al. Analysis of families in the multiple autoimmune disease genetics consortium (MADGC) collection: the PTPN22 620W allele associates with multiple autoimmune phenotypes. *Am J Hum Genet* 2005;76:561–71.

16. Smyth D, Cooper JD, Collins JE et al. Replication of an association between the lymphoid tyrosine phosphatase locus (LYP/PTPN22) with type 1 diabetes, and evidence for its role as a general autoimmunity locus. *Diabetes* 2004;53:3020–3.

17. Velaga MR, Wilson V, Jennings CE et al. The codon 620 tryptophan allele of the lymphoid tyrosine phosphatase (LYP) gene is a major determinant of Graves' disease. *J Clin Endocrinol Metab* 2004;89:5862–5.

18. Skorka A, Bednarczuk T, Bar-Andziak E et al. Lymphoid tyrosine phosphatase (PTPN22/LYP) variant and Graves' disease in a Polish population: association and gene dose-dependent correlation with age of onset. *Clin Endocrinol (Oxf)* 2005;62:679–82.

19. Suzuki A, Yamada R, Chang X et al. Functional haplotypes of PADI4, encoding citrullinating enzyme peptidylarginine deiminase 4, are associated with rheumatoid arthritis. *Nat Genet* 2003;34: 395–402.

20. Ikari K, Kuwahara M, Nakamura T et al. Association between PADI4 and rheumatoid arthritis: a replication study. *Arthritis Rheum* 2005;52:3054–7.

21. Barton A, Bowes J, Eyre S et al. A functional haplotype of the PADI4 gene associated with rheumatoid arthritis in a Japanese population is not associated in a United Kingdom population. *Arthritis Rheum* 2004; 50:1117–21.

22. Martinez A, Valdivia A, Pascual-Salcedo D et al. PADI4 polymorphisms are not associated with rheumatoid arthritis in the Spanish population. *Rheumatology (Oxford)* 2005;44:1263–6.

23. Remmers E, Plenge R, Le J et al. Comprehensive analysis of sequence variation in the peptidyl arginine deiminase type IV gene (PADI4) suggests a novel intronic variant is associated with rheumatoid arthritis in the North American Caucasian population. *Arthritis Rheum* 2006; in press.

24. Kochi Y, Yamada R, Suzuki A et al. A functional variant in FCRL3, encoding Fc receptor-like 3, is associated with rheumatoid arthritis and several autoimmunities. *Nat Genet* 2005;37:478–85.

25. Tokuhiro S, Yamada R, Chang X et al. An intronic SNP in a RUNX1 binding site of SLC22A4, encoding an organic cation transporter, is associated with rheumatoid arthritis. *Nat Genet* 2003;35:341–8.

26. Swanberg M, Lidman O, Padyukov L et al. MHC2TA is associated with differential MHC molecule expression and susceptibility to rheumatoid arthritis, multiple sclerosis and myocardial infarction. *Nat Genet* 2005;37:486–94.

B-lymphocyte depletion in rheumatic diseases

YK Onno Teng MD and Ferdinand C Breedveld MD PhD
Department of Rheumatology, Leiden University Medical Center,
The Netherlands

Rheumatic diseases, including rheumatoid arthritis (RA), systemic lupus erythematosus (SLE) and Wegener's granulomatosis, share a common immune abnormality characterized by the production of autoantibodies.[1] Since their discovery more than 50 years ago,[2,3] these circulating autoantibodies have provided the key argument that B lymphocytes play a pivotal role in the pathophysiology of rheumatic diseases.

Role of B lymphocytes in rheumatic diseases

B lymphocytes can contribute in several ways to the development of rheumatic diseases:

- as precursors of (auto)antibody-secreting plasma cells
- as (auto)antigen-presenting cells.

  In addition, when activated, they:
- produce cytokines (e.g. tumor necrosis factor alpha [TNFα]) that may influence the function of antigen-presenting dendritic cells
- express costimulatory molecules that can be essential for the evolution of T effector cells.[4]

Autoantibodies

Autoantibodies are typically directed against several components of the human body, such as nuclear antigens, double-stranded (ds)DNA and, in the case of rheumatoid factors, the 'constant region' or 'Fc' of immunoglobulins.

The exact role of autoantibodies in the pathophysiology of rheumatic diseases is still unclear – early clinical studies that eliminated autoantibodies by plasmapheresis or absorption did not improve outcomes. In this respect, the efficacy of B-lymphocyte-depleting strategies in rheumatic diseases suggests that the cellular function of B lymphocytes is important in maintaining disease activity.

B-lymphocyte depletion is achieved by using monoclonal antibodies directed against membrane proteins, including CD20 (rituximab, HuMax-CD20) and CD22 (epratuzumab), which are only present on B lymphocytes. These therapeutic agents are categorized as 'biologics' (medical preparations made from living organisms and their products).

Depleting B lymphocytes

Research has focused on the first approved (for lymphoma) B-lymphocyte-depleting agent, rituximab, which targets the CD20 membrane protein. It is generally accepted that the membrane-bound CD20 protein regulates ion influx at calcium channels.[5] It is found specifically on the membrane of B lymphocytes, but is not expressed on stem cells nor on terminally differentiated plasma cells.

Rituximab is already in use as a therapeutic agent in hematologic practice for the treatment of B-cell non-Hodgkin's lymphomas. In contrast, other B-cell-depleting agents, such as epratuzumab, have only recently been studied in hematologic patients, so phase I and II clinical studies in patients with rheumatic conditions have only recently started.

Clinical studies with rituximab

Several clinical trials have been published in which rituximab has been used to treat patients with RA, SLE, Wegener's granulomatosis and Sjögren's syndrome. Except for the RA trial, these have all been phase I and II studies, illustrating that B-cell-depletion therapy is a novel and emerging treatment strategy in the practice of rheumatology.

In the treatment of RA, rituximab has already been used 'off label' by many rheumatologists for patients with severe, therapy-refractory disease.

In rheumatoid arthritis. It has frequently been reported that RA patients with circulating autoantibodies, such as rheumatoid factor, have a more progressive disease and a worse prognosis.[6,7] More recently, it has been shown that autoantibodies against cyclic citrullinated peptides (CCPs) are very specific for RA,[8] and that CCP autoantibodies might be a cause of the chronic inflammation experienced by patients with RA.[9] Therefore, it was hypothesized that depletion of B cells would have a positive effect on reducing the disease symptoms in patients with RA.

Following several open-label studies of rituximab treatment that showed promising improvements in patients with RA, Edwards et al. conducted a randomized, placebo-controlled, multicenter trial to assess the efficacy of rituximab as a single agent or in combination therapy with methotrexate or cyclophosphamide. The study assessed 160 patients with RA, and compared the rituximab regimens with methotrexate alone.[10] The primary endpoint was defined as an ACR50 response (i.e. a 50% or greater improvement in the signs and symptoms of RA, as defined by the American College of Rheumatology [ACR]) within 24 weeks. In this pivotal trial, 33% of the patients treated with rituximab alone achieved an ACR50 response, compared with 13% in the methotrexate group. The differences were even larger when combination therapy was used: 43% and 41% of patients achieved an ACR50 response when treated with rituximab in combination with methotrexate and cyclophosphamide, respectively. Naturally, more patients achieved an ACR20 response (20% improvement) in this trial, the main results of which are summarized in Figure 1. Treatment with rituximab, particularly when combined with methotrexate, remained more efficacious than methotrexate alone for at least 1 year. In addition, extension studies showed sustained benefit from a single course of rituximab for up to 2 years. Similar efficacy has been achieved with subsequent treatment courses of rituximab.[11,12]

Further evidence for the efficacy of rituximab in RA comes from the Dose-ranging Assessment iNternational Clinical Evaluation of Rituximab in rheumatoid arthritis (DANCER) trial, which examined the efficacy of different doses of rituximab (500 mg b.d.

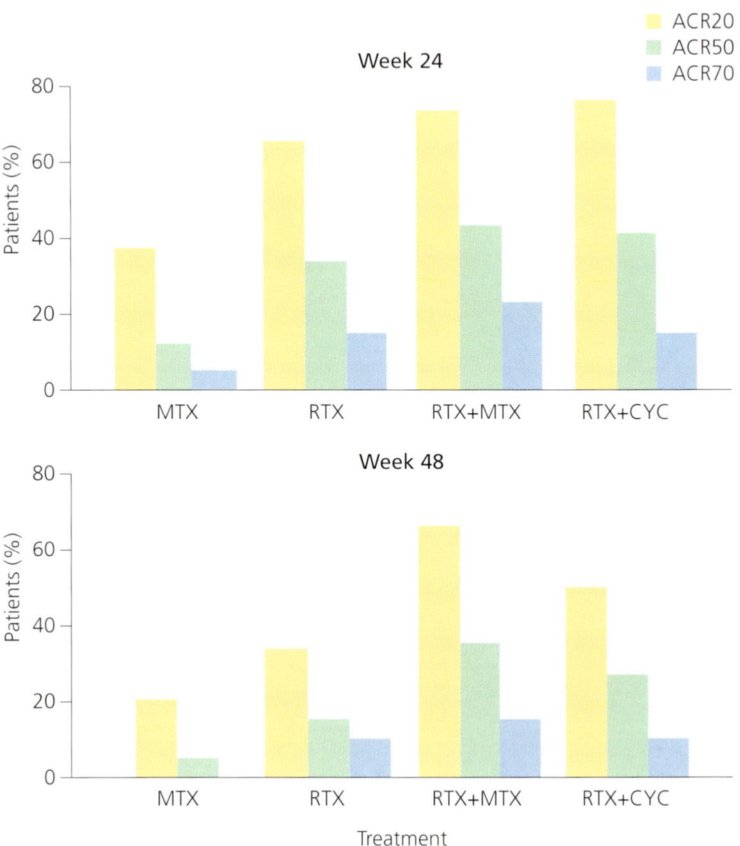

Figure 1 Percentage of patients (n = 160) with rheumatoid arthritis achieving a 20% (ACR20), 50% (ACR50) or 70% (ACR70) improvement in response according to American College of Rheumatology criteria, after single or combination treatment with rituximab compared with methotrexate monotherapy. (Note that patients with an ACR20 response are also included in the ACR50 and ACR70 data; likewise, those with an ACR50 response are included again in the ACR70 data.) CYC, cyclophosphamide; MTX, methotrexate; RTX, rituximab. Adapted from Edwards et al.[10]

vs 1000 mg b.d. on days 1 and 15) and glucocorticoids in combination with stable doses of methotrexate.[13] This trial affirmed the previous positive effects of rituximab on RA disease activity.

There was no difference in primary outcomes (ACR20 and ACR50 responses) between medium (500 mg) and high (1000 mg) doses of rituximab. However, using more stringent outcome measures (e.g. ACR70 response or remission defined by disease activity score) a trend in favor of high doses was observed. Furthermore, more patients developed circulating human antichimeric antibodies (HACA) when treated with medium doses (4.9% vs 2.7%).

The DANCER study also demonstrated that corticosteroids administered during the first 15 days of therapy (around the doses of rituximab) did not contribute to efficacy. Intravenous methylprednisolone (100 mg i.v. before rituximab infusions) ameliorated 'cytokine release' symptoms in many patients, but there was no added benefit of oral corticosteroids on days 2 to 14 in between infusions. More recently, the Randomized Evaluation oF Long-term Efficacy of rituXimab (REFLEX) study also showed rituximab to be highly effective in patients with RA who had experienced an inadequate response to one or more TNF-blocking agent.[14]

In systemic lupus erythematosus. Autoantibodies directed at dsDNA are typical in patients with SLE. Furthermore, an increase in concentration of these circulating autoantibodies is known to be associated with a reactivation of disease symptoms in many patients. Because of this direct association of anti-dsDNA antibodies with disease activity, SLE is also seen as a classic B-lymphocyte-mediated autoimmune disease.[15]

Randomized clinical trials analyzing the efficacy of rituximab in patients with SLE are being conducted. These studies are based on the promising results of two small, open-label, uncontrolled trials that evaluated 24 and 13 patients with SLE. Rituximab had a positive effect on both the SLE Disease Activity Index (SLEDAI) and the British Isles Lupus Assessment Group (BILAG) disease activity index in 95% and 69% of patients in these two studies, respectively. Anti dsDNA antibody levels significantly decreased after therapy, even to undetectable values, and the complement profile of the patients improved.[16,17]

Taken together, these results suggest that rituximab has a positive effect in patients with previously refractory SLE. Still, it is necessary to await the results of larger, ongoing trials to confirm these positive outcomes. Thereafter, it will be necessary to develop optimal treatment strategies and indications for the use of rituximab in patients with SLE.

In Wegener's granulomatosis. Wegener's granulomatosis is a primary systemic small-vessel vasculitis, which is associated with circulating antineutrophil cytoplasmic antibodies (ANCA). These react with either neutrophil proteinase 3 (PR3) or myeloperoxidase (MPO). It has been shown that the number of activated B lymphocytes in peripheral blood is linked to disease activity in patients with Wegener's granulomatosis and that a rise in ANCA titers can predict relapses in many patients.[18,19]

Suggestions that rituximab may be effective in Wegener's granulomatosis come from two recently published pilot studies. In one of these two prospective, open-label trials, 9 out of 10 patients with Wegener's granulomatosis achieved a stable clinical remission during follow-up and could safely be tapered from corticosteroid treatment without relapse.[20] In the second study, 7 out of 9 ANCA-positive vasculitis patients achieved a similar remission.[21] The disease activity was documented by the internationally accepted Birmingham Vasculitis Activity Score (BVAS).

Although these results look promising, no definitive conclusions can be drawn from the limited data available. Nevertheless, these findings have led to the initiation of a phase III trial in patients with Wegener's granulomatosis, the recruitment phase of which started recently.

In Sjögren's syndrome. The presence of rheumatoid factor, anti-SSA and anti-SSB antibodies and hypergammaglobulinemia in patients with Sjögren's syndrome strongly suggests that B-lymphocyte hyperactivity is involved in the pathophysiology of the disease. Because there is no evidence-based intervention therapy for Sjögren's syndrome, and there are no validated disease activity criteria, the assessment of the efficacy of new treatment modalities presents a challenge. Until now, only one open-label, phase II study has been published. In this study, in which 15 patients with Sjögren's syndrome were treated with rituximab, both the objective and subjective parameters for disease improved significantly.[22] Interestingly, salivary gland function in these patients only improved if they had substantial residual exocrine gland function. This supports the hypothesis that patients with Sjögren's syndrome might benefit from early treatment.

Safety. Rituximab has been used in general hematologic practice for more than 10 years. Long-term safety is well established in these patients, with no increase in the incidence of infection; most infections were typical of those commonly found in normal hosts.[23] Long-term safety data for patients with rheumatic conditions are scarce, and conclusions can only be drawn in relation to the short-term adverse events. Most of the side effects occur during intravenous administration; they tend to be mild (e.g. nausea, fever, headache, myalgia and the 'cytokine release' syndrome). As mentioned previously, the DANCER study concluded that the administration of corticosteroids before infusion of rituximab did not influence efficacy, but did reduce the incidence of infusion-related side effects – from 46% to 32% at the first infusion.[24]

Time to repletion. Depletion of B lymphocytes is a consistent and anticipated effect of rituximab treatment. The time to repletion differs for each patient and for each underlying rheumatic disease, but a mean time to repletion of 6–9 months is generally accepted.[25] Furthermore, a decrease in the concentration of serum immunoglobulins (IgG, IgM, IgA) to levels below the normal range seldom occurs. Also, notwithstanding the relatively small number of patients treated to date, the incidence of serious infectious complications is not significantly increased in patients with rheumatic diseases.[26] It is conceivable that during the period of B-cell depletion, the innate immune system provides adequate protection as a 'first line of defense'.[23]

Highlights in **B-lymphocyte depletion in rheumatic diseases** *2005–06*

WHAT'S IN?

- B-lymphocyte depletion as a new treatment modality for systemic rheumatic diseases
- Research to assess the efficacy of rituximab in different autoantibody-mediated diseases
- Development of new therapeutic biologics to induce B-lymphocyte depletion, such as epratuzumab (anti-CD22) and HuMax-CD20 (fully humanized monoclonal antibody)
- Fundamental research into the regulatory mechanisms of B lymphocytes within the immune system

WHAT'S OUT?

- Consideration of B lymphocytes as merely antibody-producing cells in rheumatic diseases

WHAT'S NEEDED?

- Studies to determine the most efficacious treatment schedule to induce long-term improvement in rheumatic disease activity

References

1. Isenberg DA, Maddison PJ, Woo P et al. *Oxford Textbook of Rheumatology*, 3rd edn. Oxford: Oxford University Press, 2004.

2. Holman HR, Kunkel HG. Affinity between the lupus erythematosus serum factor and cell nuclei and nucleoprotein. *Science* 1957;126: 162–3.

3. Rose HM, Ragan C, Pearce E et al. Differential agglutination of normal and sensitized sheep erythrocytes by sera of patients with rheumatoid arthritis. *Proc Soc Exp Biol Med* 1948;68:1–6.

4. Dorner T, Burmester GR. The role of B cells in rheumatoid arthritis: mechanisms and therapeutic targets. *Curr Opin Rheumatol* 2003;15: 246–52.

5. Ernst JA, Li H, Kim HS et al. Isolation and characterization of the B-cell marker CD20. *Biochemistry* 2005;44:15150–8.

6. Uhlig T, Smedstad LM, Vaglum P et al. The course of rheumatoid arthritis and predictors of psychological, physical and radiographic outcome after 5 years of follow-up. *Rheumatology (Oxford)* 2000;39:732–41.

7. Forslind K, Ahlmen M, Eberhardt K et al. Prediction of radiological outcome in early rheumatoid arthritis in clinical practice: role of antibodies to citrullinated peptides (anti-CCP). *Ann Rheum Dis* 2004;63:1090–5.

8. van Gaalen FA, Visser H, Huizinga TW. A comparison of the diagnostic accuracy and prognostic value of the first and second anti cyclic citrullinated peptides (CCP1 and CCP2) autoantibody tests for rheumatoid arthritis. *Ann Rheum Dis* 2005;64:1510–12.

9. van Gaalen F, Ioan-Facsinay A, Huizinga TW, Toes RE. The devil in the details: the emerging role of anticitrulline autoimmunity in rheumatoid arthritis. *J Immunol* 2005;175:5575–80.

10. Edwards JC, Szczepanski L, Szechinski J et al. Efficacy of B-cell-targeted therapy with rituximab in patients with rheumatoid arthritis. *N Engl J Med* 2004;350:2572–81.

11. Pavelka K, Emery P, Filipowicz-Sosnowska A et al. Efficacy and safety following repeated courses of rituximab in patients with active rheumatoid arthritis. *Proceedings of EULAR 2005. Vienna, Austria, 8–11 June, 2005.* Abstr [SAT0080]. www.abstracts2view.com/eular

12. Strand V, Balbir-Gurman A, Pavelka K et al. Two-year improvements in physical function reflect sustained benefit in rheumatoid arthritis patients receiving a single course of rituximab with methotrexate. *Proceedings of EULAR 2005. Vienna, Austria, 8–11 June, 2005.* Abstr [THU0329]. www.abstracts2view.com/eular

13. van Vollenhoven RF, Schechtman J, Szczepanski LJ et al. Safety and tolerability of rituximab in patients with moderate to severe rheumatoid arthritis: results from the DANCER study. *Proceedings of ACR 2005. San Diego, USA, 12–17 November 2005.* Abstr 1922. www.rheumatology.org/annual/abstracts/search.asp

14. Cohen SB, Greenwald M, Dougados MR et al. Efficacy and safety of rituximab in active RA patients who experienced an inadequate response to one or more anti-TNFα therapies (REFLEX study). *Proceedings of ACR 2005. San Diego, USA, 12–17 November 2005.* Abstr 1830. www.rheumatology.org/annual/abstracts/search.asp

15. Janeway CA, Travers P, Walport M, Shlochick M. *Immunobiology: The Immune System in Health and Disease,* 6th edn. New York: Garland Science, 2005.

16. Leandro MJ, Cambridge G, Edwards JC et al. B-cell depletion in the treatment of patients with systemic lupus erythematosus: a longitudinal analysis of 24 patients. *Rheumatology (Oxford)* 2005;44: 1542–5.

17. Gottenberg JE, Guillevin L, Lambotte O et al. Tolerance and short term efficacy of rituximab in 43 patients with systemic autoimmune diseases. *Ann Rheum Dis* 2005;64: 913–20.

18. Popa ER, Stegeman CA, Bos NA et al. Differential B- and T-cell activation in Wegener's granulomatosis. *J Allergy Clin Immunol* 1999;103:885–94.

19. Boomsma MM, Stegeman CA, vander Leij MJ et al. Prediction of relapses in Wegener's granulomatosis by measurement of antineutrophil cytoplasmic antibody levels: a prospective study. *Arthritis Rheum* 2000;43:2025–33.

20. Keogh KA, Ytterberg SR, Fervenza FC et al. Rituximab for refractory Wegener's granulomatosis: report of a prospective, open-label pilot trial. *Am J Respir Crit Care Med* 2006;173:180–7.

21. Eriksson P. Nine patients with anti-neutrophil cytoplasmic antibody-positive vasculitis successfully treated with rituximab. *J Intern Med* 2005;257:540–8.

22. Pijpe J, van Imhoff GW, Spijkervet FK et al. Rituximab treatment in patients with primary Sjögren's syndrome: an open-label phase II study. *Arthritis Rheum* 2005;52:2740–50.

23. McLaughlin P. Rituximab: perspective on single agent experience, and future directions in combination trials. *Crit Rev Oncol Hematol* 2001;40:3–16.

24. Fleischmann RM, Emery P, Filipowicz-Sosnowska A et al. Coadministration of glucocorticoids does not influence efficacy of, but reduces infusion reactions to, rituximab in rheumatoid arthritis: results from the DANCER study. *Proceedings of EULAR 2005. Vienna, Austria, 8–11 June, 2005.* Abstr [SAT 0077]. www.abstracts2view.com/eular

25. Edwards JC, Cambridge G. Prospects for B-cell-targeted therapy in autoimmune disease. *Rheumatology (Oxford)* 2005;44:151–6.

26. Gorman C, Leandro M, Isenberg D. B cell depletion in autoimmune disease. *Arthritis Res Ther* 2003;5(suppl 4):S17–21.

Interleukin–15

J Alastair Gracie PhD and Iain B McInnes FRCP PhD
Division of Immunology, Infection and Inflammation, University of Glasgow, UK

Substantial benefits have been achieved in a proportion of patients with rheumatoid arthritis (RA) by targeting tumor necrosis factor-α (TNFα).[1] However, there remains considerable unmet clinical need, as a significant proportion of patients who receive this therapy do not experience acceptable improvement.

Better understanding of the disease processes in RA synovitis has identified novel potential targets among those cytokines that display pro-inflammatory activity. Here we focus on one, interleukin-15 (IL-15), briefly reviewing its structure and function. We also consider recent data supporting the notion that IL-15 blockade offers therapeutic potential for both partial- and non-responders to TNFα-blocking agents and/or in synergy with existing targeted approaches.

Structure and function

IL-15 is an innate response, 14-15-kDa, four-α-helix cytokine with structural similarities to IL-2.[2,3] IL-15 mRNA is relatively stable and is found in numerous normal human tissues and cell types, including activated monocytes, dendritic cells and fibroblasts.[3] In contrast, protein expression is far more restricted, reflecting tight regulatory control of translation and secretion.[4,5] IL-15 mRNA has two forms, with different leader sequences that, in turn, promote the localization of the protein within the cytosol or the membrane, or promote secretion.[5]

The intracellular activities of IL-15 are unknown. The sequence of IL-15 contains a putative transmembrane domain that, in part, explains membrane expression. Cell membrane expression of IL-15 may be crucial for mediating its extracellular function, and partly explains why it is difficult to detect soluble IL-15 in biological systems. Membrane-bound and extracellularly secreted IL-15 functions by binding via a widely distributed heterotrimeric receptor (IL-15R), which consists of a β-chain (shared with IL-2), a common γ-chain and a unique α-chain (IL-15α).[5] While IL-15 binds to the βγ-chain heterodimer with intermediate affinity, IL-15 binds to the IL-15Rα with high affinity (10^{11} M^{-1}) and has a slow rate of dissociation from the receptor (off-rate). This has proven useful in studies using in-vitro and in-vivo models to determine the role of IL-15 in inflammation and host defense.

Indeed, the high affinity and slow off-rate make IL-15Rα in soluble form a useful and specific inhibitor in biological systems. IL-15Rα is widely distributed; it is expressed on many immune cells, including T cells, natural killer (NK) and natural killer T (NKT) cells, B cells and macrophages.[6] In addition, IL-15Rα mRNA is expressed in a number of non-lymphoid cell types and organs such as vascular endothelium, spleen, skeletal muscle, heart and lungs.

Like IL-2, the IL-15Rαβγ complex signals through Janus kinases (JAKs) 1 and 3 and signal transducer and activator of transcription (STAT)-3 and -5.[6,7] Additional signaling through src-related tyrosine kinases and Ras/Raf/mitogen-activated protein kinase to fos/jun activation has also been proposed. The receptor complex is unusual in that the IL-15Rα component may be expressed either on the same cell as βγ chains (*cis*), or on an adjacent cell (*trans*).[8] Indeed, it has been shown that activated monocytes can present *in trans* via the stably expressed IL-15/IL-15Rα cell surface complex to $CD8^+$ T cells, which themselves only express the lower affinity βγ receptor complex as shown in Figure 1.

It has recently been shown that activated monocytes can express membrane-anchored IL-15 directly on their cell surfaces independent of IL-15Rα.[9] This leads to cellular activation, signal pathway activation and migration, suggesting that IL-15 can itself act as a signaling receptor – so-called ‘reverse signaling’.

Tables 1 and 2 describe the bioactivities of IL-15, and diseases in which IL-15 is implicated in the pathology.

Key biological effects

IL-15 is found in a broad range of normal human tissues and cell types, including activated monocytes, dendritic cells, myocytes, adipocytes and fibroblasts.[3,5]

As predicted by the cellular distribution of its receptor, IL-15 mediates broad functional effects. It has a critical role in the development, activation and maintenance of NK and T cells, particularly of memory phenotype, protecting them from apoptosis.[10,11] IL-15 also mediates the recruitment and activation of neutrophils[12] and B cells, and promotes the survival of fibroblast-like synoviocytes and vascular endothelial cells.[13] Particularly

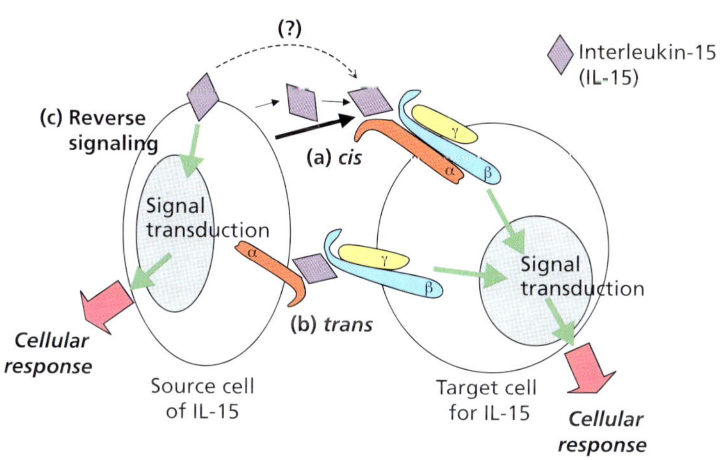

Figure 1 Three models for IL-15/IL-15R engagement. (a) The traditional model suggests that IL-15 is released from the source cell and binds to the IL-15R heterotrimer on the target cell, inducing signal transduction and cellular response (*cis*). (b) As suggested by Dubois et al.,[8] IL-15 can be presented by IL-15Rα on the source cell to the βγ heterodimer on the target cell, again inducing a cellular response (*trans*). (c) A third mechanism, suggested by Budagian et al.,[9] proposes that membrane-bound, biologically active IL-15 induces 'reverse signaling', whereby the cell is self-activated. Finally, it is possible that such membrane-bound IL-15 binds to the IL-15R heterotrimer on the adjacent cell, thereby inducing a cellular response.

TABLE 1
Key bioactivities of interleukin-15

Cell	Biological effect
Neutrophil	Neutrophil activation; induces rearrangements of cytoskeletal structure; delays apoptosis; enhances chemotaxis, phagocytosis, respiratory burst and cytokine release
T cell	TH1/TH2 maturation; enhances migration, activation, cytokine release, cytotoxicity and T-cell memory maintenance (CD8$^+$ compartment)
Natural killer (NK) cell	NK-cell maturation; activation; cytokine release; cytotoxicity
B cell	Isotype switching; immunoglobulin production
Macrophage	Enhances cytokine expression and adhesion molecule expression
Dendritic cell	Activation; co-stimulation; enhances cytokine release
Endothelial cell	Enhances activation/migration; retards apoptosis
Fibroblast-like synoviocyte	Enhances activation/proliferation; retards apoptosis
Osteoclast	Enhances maturation; upregulates calcitonin receptor

important functions reside in the regulation of dendritic cell/T cell interactions.[14,15] Finally, pro-angiogenic effects have been proposed.[16]

However, such activities are not without consequence. It has been proposed that, by preventing IL-2 from promoting activation-induced cell death, IL-15 inhibits self-tolerance by allowing autoreactive CD8$^+$ memory T cells to survive.[17,18]

TABLE 2

Diseases in which a pathological role for interleukin-15 is implicated

- Rheumatoid arthritis
- Psoriasis
- Pulmonary inflammation (chronic obstructive pulmonary disease, sarcoidosis, pulmonary tuberculosis)
- Inflammatory bowel disease
- Multiple sclerosis
- Autoimmune diabetes
- Celiac disease
- Transplant rejection
- Cardiovascular disease
- Leukemia

Evidence for a role in inflammatory arthritis

Relevant expression and biological activities of IL-15 in the context of inflammatory arthritis have now been well characterized.

- IL-15 is detected in inflamed synovial membrane and synovial fluid, and at lower concentrations in some serum samples, from patients with RA, psoriatic arthritis, juvenile idiopathic arthritis (JIA) and reactive arthritis. Detection has been via enzyme-linked immunosorbent assay (ELISA), receptor capture assay, Western blotting, reverse transcriptase–polymerase chain reaction (RT-PCR) and Taqman PCR. Relevant receptor components, namely IL-15Rα, IL-15/2 receptor β and the common γ chain, are also present.[19–21]
- Serum levels of IL-15 rise progressively with the duration of RA.[22] IL-15 levels in JIA correlate with levels of C-reactive protein.[23]
- IL-15 promotes the pro-inflammatory release of chemokines and cytokines, including TNFα and IL-1β.[24]
- IL-15 enhances synovial T-cell proliferation and the subsequent cognate interaction of T cells with macrophages.[24] IL-15 promotes

neutrophil activation, NK-cell granule release and endothelial-cell activation/migration. IL-15 and TNF together promote expression of NKG2D on potentially autoreactive $CD4^+$ $CD28^-$ RA T cells.[25]

- In the collagen-induced arthritis rodent model, the soluble IL-15Rα chain reduces clinically evident inflammation and histological evidence of articular destruction, whether given prophylactically or after the disease has become established.[26]

Targeting in clinical trials

A number of therapeutic agents that inhibit IL-15 action have been, or will shortly be, introduced allowing the specific targeting of IL-15. These include soluble forms of the IL-15Rα,[26] a mutant IL-15 that acts as a competitive antagonist,[27] and a small molecule inhibitor of IL-15 receptor signaling. However, first to be assessed by clinical trial have been specific neutralizing antibodies, targeting either IL-15 itself or the βγ chains of the IL-15/2 receptor complex.[28,29]

A fully human immunoglobulin (Ig)G_1 monoclonal antibody (AMG714) has been developed that is capable of binding not only soluble but also membrane-bound IL-15. AMG714 (previously HuMax-IL15) neutralizes soluble and membrane-bound IL-15 in vitro. In a dose-ascending, placebo-controlled phase I study, AMG714 was administered to patients with RA (n = 30) over 12 weeks. Patients received a randomized, controlled, single dose of AMG714 (0.5–8 mg/kg) at week 0 followed by open-label, weekly doses from weeks 4 to 7. IL-15 neutralization was well tolerated and improvements in disease activity were observed, with 63%, 38% and 25% of patients demonstrating a 20%, 50% and 70% improvement at week 8, respectively, according to American College of Rheumatology (ACR) criteria.[28] This study was, however, small and not adequately controlled. A subsequent dose-finding study was performed in which patients received increasing doses of anti-IL-15 antibody for 3 months. An interim analysis indicated satisfactory tolerance compared with placebo, and ACR20 improvements were observed in approximately 60% of recipients receiving higher doses of AMG714. No significant alterations in the levels of circulating leukocyte subsets, including NK cells and $CD8^+$ memory T cells,

Highlights in **interleukin-15** *2005–06*

WHAT'S IN?

- Clinical trials of interleukin-15 (IL-15) blockade
- Recognition of a potential role for IL-15 in tolerance breakdown
- The concept of 'reverse signaling' for IL-15

WHAT'S OUT?

- The belief that tumor necrosis factor-α is the only therapeutically targetable cytokine in rheumatoid arthritis (RA)

WHAT'S NEEDED?

- Research to determine the optimal targeting modality for IL-15 blockade
- Research to determine the optimal kinetics for IL-15 blockade
- Studies of IL-15 blockade in inflammatory diseases other than RA

were observed. Larger, confirmatory studies are now required to facilitate proper interpretation of these data, and, at this stage, IL-15 should not be considered a validated therapeutic target.

Key outstanding questions

Early encouraging clinical studies in which IL-15 has been neutralized now require confirmation. The optimal kinetics of IL-15 blockade have not yet been achieved. In particular, the potential role in tolerance maintenance offers intriguing therapeutic possibilities. IL-15:Fc fusion protein (a competitive antagonist to IL-15) suppresses delayed-type hypersensitivity in rodent models and delays cardiac transplant rejection.[27]

Therefore, the key areas of focus in IL-15 research are:

- the optimal targeting modality
- the precise timing of IL-15 neutralization
- its comparability in patients with partial or absent responses to existing biological agents, especially TNFα blockade
- its expression across a range of rheumatic disorders, and characterization of its therapeutic utility therein.

References

1. Feldmann M, Maini RN. Lasker Clinical Medical Research Award. TNF defined as a therapeutic target for rheumatoid arthritis and other autoimmune diseases. *Nat Med* 2003;9:1245–50.

2. Bamford RN, Battiata AP, Burton JD et al. Interleukin (IL) 15/IL-T production by the adult T-cell leukemia cell line HuT-102 is associated with a human T-cell lymphotrophic virus type I region/IL-15 fusion message that lacks many upstream AUGs that normally attenuates IL-15 mRNA translation. *Proc Natl Acad Sci USA* 1996; 93:2897–902.

3. Grabstein KH, Eisenman J, Shanebeck K et al. Cloning of a T cell growth factor that interacts with the beta chain of the interleukin-2 receptor. *Science* 1994;264:965–8.

4. Fehniger TA, Caligiuri MA. Interleukin 15: biology and relevance to human disease. *Blood* 2001;97:14–32.

5. Waldmann TA, Tagaya Y. The multifaceted regulation of interleukin-15 expression and the role of this cytokine in NK cell differentiation and host response to intracellular pathogens. *Annu Rev Immunol* 1999;17:19–49.

6. Giri JG, Kumaki S, Ahdieh M et al. Identification and cloning of a novel IL-15 binding protein that is structurally related to the alpha chain of the IL-2 receptor. *EMBO J* 1995;14:3654–63.

7. Waldmann T, Tagaya Y, Bamford R. Interleukin-2, interleukin-15, and their receptors. *Int Rev Immunol* 1998;16:205–26.

8. Dubois S, Mariner J, Waldmann TA, Tagaya Y. IL-15Ralpha recycles and presents IL-15 in trans to neighboring cells. *Immunity* 2002;17:537–47.

9. Budagian V, Bulanova E, Orinska Z et al. Reverse signaling through membrane-bound interleukin-15. *J Biol Chem* 2004;279:42192–201.

10. Lodolce JP, Burkett PR, Koka RM et al. Regulation of lymphoid homeostasis by interleukin-15. *Cytokine Growth Factor Rev* 2002;13:429–39.

11. Schluns KS, Lefrancois L. Cytokine control of memory T-cell development and survival. *Nat Rev Immunol* 2003;3:269–79.

12. Girard D, Paquet ME, Paquin R, Beaulieu AD. Differential effects of interleukin-15 (IL-15) and IL-2 on human neutrophils: modulation of phagocytosis, cytoskeleton rearrangement, gene expression, and apoptosis by IL-15. *Blood* 1996;88:3176–84.

13. Yang L, Thornton S, Grom AA. Interleukin-15 inhibits sodium nitroprusside-induced apoptosis of synovial fibroblasts and vascular endothelial cells. *Arthritis Rheum* 2002;46:3010–14.

14. Jonuleit H, Wiedemann K, Muller G et al. Induction of IL-15 messenger RNA and protein in human blood-derived dendritic cells: a role for IL-15 in attraction of T cells. *J Immunol* 1997;158: 2610–15.

15. Mohamadzadeh M, Berard F, Essert G et al. Interleukin 15 skews monocyte differentiation into dendritic cells with features of Langerhans cells. *J Exp Med* 2001;194:1013–20.

16. Angiolillo AL, Kanegane H, Sgadari C et al. Interleukin-15 promotes angiogenesis in vivo. *Biochem Biophys Res Commun* 1997;233:231–7.

17. Waldmann TA, Dubois S, Tagaya Y. Contrasting roles of IL-2 and IL-15 in the life and death of lymphocytes: implications for immunotherapy. *Immunity* 2001; 14:105–10.

18. Zhang X, Sun S, Hwang I et al. Potent and selective stimulation of memory-phenotype CD8$^+$ T cells in vivo by IL-15. *Immunity* 1998;8: 591–9.

19. McInnes IB, al-Mughales J, Field M et al. The role of interleukin-15 in T-cell migration and activation in rheumatoid arthritis. *Nat Med* 1996;2:175–82.

20. Kotake S, Schumacher HR Jr, Yarboro CH et al. In vivo gene expression of type 1 and type 2 cytokines in synovial tissues from patients in early stages of rheumatoid, reactive, and undifferentiated arthritis. *Proc Assoc Am Physicians* 1997;109:286–301.

21. Harada S, Yamamura M, Okamoto H et al. Production of interleukin-7 and interleukin-15 by fibroblast-like synoviocytes from patients with rheumatoid arthritis. *Arthritis Rheum* 1999;42:1508–16.

22. Gonzalez-Alvaro I, Ortiz AM, Garcia-Vicuna R et al. Increased serum levels of interleukin-15 in rheumatoid arthritis with long-term disease. *Clin Exp Rheumatol* 2003;21:639–42.

23. Smolewska E, Brozik H, Smolewski P et al. Apoptosis of peripheral blood lymphocytes in patients with juvenile idiopathic arthritis. *Ann Rheum Dis* 2003;62:761–3.

24. McInnes IB, Leung BP, Sturrock RD et al. Interleukin-15 mediates T cell-dependent regulation of tumor necrosis factor-alpha production in rheumatoid arthritis. *Nat Med* 1997;3:189–95.

25. Groh V, Bruhl A, El-Gabalawy H et al. Stimulation of T cell autoreactivity by anomalous expression of NKG2D and its MIC ligands in rheumatoid arthritis. *Proc Natl Acad Sci USA* 2003;100: 9452–7.

26. Ruchatz H, Leung BP, Wei XQ et al. Soluble IL-15 receptor alpha-chain administration prevents murine collagen-induced arthritis: a role for IL-15 in development of antigen-induced immunopathology. *J Immunol* 1998;160:5654–60.

27. Zheng XX, Sanchez-Fueyo A, Sho M et al. Favorably tipping the balance between cytopathic and regulatory T cells to create transplantation tolerance. *Immunity* 2003;19:503–14.

28. Baslund B, Tvede N, Danneskiold-Samsoe B et al. Targeting interleukin-15 in patients with rheumatoid arthritis: a proof-of-concept study. *Arthritis Rheum* 2005;52:2686–92.

29. Morris JC, Janik JE, White JD et al. Preclinical and phase I clinical trial of blockade of IL-15 using Mikbeta1 monoclonal antibody in T cell large granular lymphocyte leukemia. *Proc Natl Acad Sci USA* 2006;103:401–6.

Primary Sjögren's syndrome

Simon J Bowman PhD FRCP
Rheumatology Department, University Hospital Birmingham, UK

Sjögren's syndrome is characterized by focal lymphocytic infiltration of the exocrine glands, and is associated particularly with dryness of the eyes and mouth.[1] It occurs as a primary disorder (primary Sjögren's syndrome [PSS]) or secondary to other rheumatic diseases (e.g. rheumatoid arthritis [RA] or systemic lupus erythematosus [SLE]). There is a strong female bias, and most recent studies suggest a prevalence among young women of 0.2–0.6% for PSS. In total, 70% of patients with PSS have anti-Ro (also known as anti-SSA) and/or anti-La autoantibodies, often in association with hypergammaglobulinemia; these patients are at greatest risk of systemic involvement. B-cell hyperactivity may also contribute to the 44-fold increased risk of B-cell lymphoma found in patients with PSS.

Classification and diagnosis

The field has been complicated by the use of a number of different classification criteria. This has made comparison between publications difficult and is confusing in clinical practice. The key development in recent years has been the use of the American–European criteria (Tables 1 and 2)[2] in most studies. Although these are technically classification rather than diagnostic criteria, they are useful as diagnostic criteria for most patients in clinical practice.

Clinical features and therapy

Sicca features are often inadequately treated. Simple measures and advice are critical, but are only helpful if patients and their physicians know how to access this information (e.g. the recently published guidelines of the British Sjögren's Syndrome Association at www.bssa.uk.net).

TABLE 1

The European classification criteria screening questions for dry eye and mouth symptoms

I. Ocular symptoms: a positive response to at least one of the following three questions:

- Have you had daily, persistent, troublesome dry eyes for > 3 months?
- Do you have recurrent sensation of sand or gravel in the eyes?
- Do you use tear substitutes > 3 times a day?

II. Oral symptoms: a positive response to at least one of the following three questions:

- Have you had a daily feeling of dry mouth for > 3 months?
- Have you had recurrently or persistently swollen salivary glands as an adult?
- Do you frequently drink liquids to aid swallowing dry food?

Adapted from Vitali et al.[2]

The key points of topical therapy are:

- saliva gels generally work better than sprays
- artificial tears should be used as often as needed
- if hypromellose is insufficient, a thicker carbomer can be substituted
- if eye drops are required more than 4–6 times a day, preservative-free drops should be used
- topical steroids are generally not advised because of the risk of infection
- topical ciclosporin drops have been shown to be effective; they are available in the USA but not in Europe.

Oral pilocarpine can stimulate saliva production. Side effects can be reduced by starting with a small dose (e.g. 2.5 mg twice daily) and increasing it slowly. An alternative, cevimeline, is, again, licensed in the USA but not in Europe.

TABLE 2

The American–European classification criteria for Sjögren's syndrome

- Symptomatic xerostomia for > 3 months: a positive response to at least one of the three European oral screening questions (see Table 1)
- Symptomatic dry eyes for > 3 months: a positive response to at least one of the three European ocular screening questions (see Table 1)
- Positive Schirmer's test (≤ 5 mm/5 minutes) or rose Bengal score (or other ocular dye score, e.g. lissamine green)
- Abnormal labial-gland biopsy (focus score ≥ 1)
- Positive result for unstimulated whole salivary flow (≤ 1.5 ml in 15 minutes) or abnormal parotid sialography or salivary scintigraphy
- Antibodies to Ro (SSA) or La (SSB), or both

Primary Sjögren's syndrome (PSS)

The presence of any four of the six items listed above indicates PSS, as long as either the labial-gland biopsy and/or anti-Ro/La antibodies are positive. Alternative criteria for PSS are three positive results out of the four objective items (ocular signs, oral signs, labial-gland biopsy, anti-Ro and/or La antibodies)

Secondary Sjögren's syndrome

In patients with another connective tissue disease, such as RA, the presence of at least one symptom item plus any two of the three objective items, excluding anti-Ro/La antibodies, may be considered as indicative of secondary Sjögren's syndrome

Exclusions

Any patient:

- with hepatitis C virus infection, acquired immunodeficiency syndrome (AIDS), pre-existing lymphoma, sarcoidosis or graft-versus-host disease
- receiving current treatment with anticholinergic drugs
- who has had previous head and neck radiation therapy

RA, rheumatoid arthritis. Adapted from Vitali et al.[2]

In patients with severe dry eyes, artificial tears can be kept on the surface of the eyes for longer by punctal occlusion, using a variety of 'plugs' to occlude the punctal openings at the inner aspects of the eyelids.

A number of novel approaches to therapy have also been reported, including autologous transfer of salivary glands to the conjunctiva to treat severe dry eyes.[3] An intraoral prosthesis that uses an electric current to stimulate saliva secretion is also under development (www.news-medical.net/?id=6598).

Research in the past 5 years has also looked at the role of aquaporins, water-channel proteins that provide a pathway for osmotic water flow across salivary and lacrimal epithelial cells. Changes in the expression or function of aquaporins may underlie the sicca symptoms in PSS. A recent paper has brought this research into the clinical arena by demonstrating that 5-aza-2'-deoxycytidine can increase expression of the gene that encodes aquaporin-5 in salivary-gland cells in vitro,[4] thus potentially increasing saliva secretion.

Gene transfer of immunomodulatory molecules[5] and the development of artificial salivary glands[6] are other novel approaches being explored.

Systemic manifestations. Patients with primary Sjögren's syndrome experience significant fatigue.[7] Arthralgias, myalgias and Raynaud's involvement are also common. Arthritis is usually mild and rarely erosive or deforming. Fibromyalgia is found in about 5% of patients, which is similar to the prevalence in RA and SLE.[7] Patients report a marked reduction in quality of life similar to that associated with RA or SLE.

Neurological involvement occurs in 20% of patients. In milder forms, such as a sensory polyneuropathy, analgesia and hydroxychloroquine may be sufficient treatment. Painful progressive sensory polyneuropathy, or sensorimotor polyneuropathy, or Sjögren's syndrome with involvement of the central nervous system are difficult to treat, as their course is unclear and no controlled trials have been performed. In a recent series of 82 patients with neurological manifestations of Sjögren's syndrome, intense immunosuppression with cyclophosphamide was needed for some patients.[8] Mycophenolate mofetil is also now being used.

Leukocytoclastic vasculitis may be associated with the presence of cryoglobulins. Patients usually have a reduced complement C4 level, and in some parts of the world this may be a feature of hepatitis C virus (HCV) infection.[9]

Studies of B-cell lymphoma (usually of mucosa-associated lymphoid tissue [MALT] origin) consistently report an approximately 44-fold increased risk in PSS, with lymphoma causing death in some patients.[10] Lymphadenopathy, parotid-gland swelling, cutaneous vasculitis, peripheral neuropathy, low-grade fever, anemia, lymphopenia and hypocomplementemia are more frequent in these patients than in the general PSS population.

At present, treatment for most patients is essentially symptomatic. Hydroxychloroquine is often used. Ciclosporin, methotrexate and azathioprine do not appear to be useful. More recently, anti-tumor-necrosis-factor (TNF) agents have been evaluated as therapeutic agents, but without great success.[11,12] New therapeutic possibilities include biologics, such as rituximab and B-lymphocyte-stimulator (BlyS)-modulating agents,[13] but formal clinical trials are needed.

Assessment tools. The development of assessment tools to quantify the clinical features of Sjögren's syndrome, including sicca features, fatigue and systemic involvement, is an area of active advances.[7,14,15] This is a prerequisite for carrying out clinical trials of new therapies for PSS, and is of particular relevance to current interest in trials of biological therapies.

Disease mechanisms

Genetics. The close association between anti-Ro/La antibodies and the human leukocyte antigen (HLA) *DR3-DQ2* haplotype is well established. More recent studies are using linkage analysis with microsatellite genetic markers and candidate gene analysis to try to identify relevant genes.[16]

Autoantibodies. The presence of anti-α-fodrin antibodies as a disease-specific marker in PSS remains very controversial.[17] The relevance to PSS of the islet cell autoantigen ICA69 is intriguing,[18] but yet to be established. Anti-muscarinic M3-receptor antibodies could be partly responsible for glandular hyposecretion in PSS, but their clinical relevance remains unclear.[19]

Viruses. It has been proposed that Sjögren's syndrome may result from an abnormal immune response to a ubiquitous virus, such as Epstein–Barr virus (EBV) or human herpesvirus (HHV)-6. Retroviruses have also been cited as potential candidates,[20] but most recent interest has focused on HCV infection, which can produce a PSS-like syndrome.[9]

Animal models

The most well-established animal model for Sjögren's syndrome is the non-obese diabetic (NOD) mouse. New mouse models reported in 2004 include the aromatase-deficient mouse, which may provide a model to study the role of estrogens in the development and/or therapy of PSS.[21]

Immunopathological features

Most recent interest has focused on dissecting the role of chemokines and their receptors in the organization of lymphoid structures in the salivary glands of patients with PSS. This is an evolving area of research and several papers have been published on this topic recently. In particular, the B-cell-attracting chemokine CXCL13, required for normal polarization of germinal centers, has been implicated as a key regulator of lymphoid neogenesis.[22] Other chemokines and receptors involved in B-cell migration and retention and T-cell-attracting chemokines and their receptors have also been studied.[23,24] B-cell activation is also a consistent immunoregulatory abnormality in Sjögren's syndrome. Of potential importance is that enhanced levels of BlyS, a B-cell growth factor belonging to the TNF family, have been demonstrated in Sjögren's syndrome.[25,26]

Highlights in **primary Sjögren's syndrome** *2005–06*

WHAT'S IN?

- The American–European criteria for classification (and diagnosis) of Sjögren's syndrome
- Proper treatment of sicca features (e.g. with oral pilocarpine) and aggressive treatment of progressive neurological involvement
- Use of disease-assessment tools and trials of anti-B-cell therapies
- The study of chemokines and B-lymphocyte stimulators, and the application of modern genetics and genomics

WHAT'S OUT?

- Other classification criteria
- Therapeutic nihilism
- Anti-tumor-necrosis-factor therapy

WHAT'S NEEDED?

- Clinical trials of systemic therapies

BlyS may potentially be involved in B-cell hyperactivity, autoantibody production, salivary-gland lymphoid organization, B-cell apoptosis and other immunoregulatory defects associated with PSS.

Another approach likely to generate new data in PSS is the application of DNA microarray technology to identify the profile of genes that are up- and downregulated in PSS salivary glands, including those encoding chemokines, TNF family members, interferons and other cytokines.[27]

References

1. Jonsson R, Bowman SJ, Gordon TP. Sjögren's Syndrome. In: Koopman WJ, Moreland LW, eds. *Arthritis and Allied Disorders (A Textbook of Rheumatology)*, 15th edn. Philadelphia: Lippincott Williams & Wilkins, 2005:1681–706.

2. Vitali C, Bombardieri S, Jonsson R et al. Classification criteria for Sjögren's syndrome: a revised version of the European criteria proposed by the American–European Consensus Group. *Ann Rheum Dis* 2002;61: 554–8.

3. Yu GY, Zhu ZH, Mao C et al. Microvascular autologous submandibular gland transfer in severe cases of keratoconjunctivitis sicca. *Int J Oral Maxillofac Surg* 2004;33:235–9.

4. Motegi K, Azuma M, Tamatani T et al. Expression of aquaporin-5 in and fluid secretion from immortalized human salivary gland ductal cells by treatment with 5-aza-2'-deoxycytidine: a possibility for improvement of xerostomia in patients with Sjögren's syndrome. *Lab Invest* 2005;85:342–53.

5. Lodde BM, Mineshiba F, Wang J et al. Effect of human vasoactive intestinal peptide gene transfer in a murine model of Sjögren's syndrome. *Ann Rheum Dis* 2006;65:195–200.

6. Tran SD, Wang J, Bandyopadhyay BC et al. Primary culture of polarized human salivary epithelial cells for use in developing an artificial salivary gland. *Tissue Eng* 2005;11:172–81.

7. Bowman SJ, Booth DA, Platts RG et al. Measurement of fatigue and discomfort in primary Sjogren's syndrome using a new questionnaire tool. *Rheumatology* 2004;43:758–64.

8. Delalande S, de Seze J, Fauchais AL et al. Neurologic manifestations in primary Sjögren syndrome: a study of 82 patients. *Medicine (Baltimore)* 2004;83:280–91.

9. Ramos-Casals M, Loustaud-Ratti V, De Vita S et al. Sjögren's syndrome associated with hepatitis C virus: a multicenter analysis of 137 cases. *Medicine (Baltimore)* 2005;84:81–9.

10. Theander E, Manthorpe R, Jacobsson LT. Mortality and causes of death in primary Sjögren's syndrome: a prospective cohort study. *Arthritis Rheum* 2004;50:1262–9.

11. Sankar V, Brennan MT, Kok MR et al. Etanercept in Sjögren's syndrome: a twelve-week randomized, double-blind, placebo-controlled pilot clinical trial. *Arthritis Rheum* 2004;50:2240–5.

12. Mariette X, Ravaud P, Steinfeld S et al. Inefficacy of infliximab in primary Sjögren's syndrome: results of the randomized, controlled Trial of Remicade In Primary Sjögren's Syndrome (TRIPSS). *Arthritis Rheum* 2004;50:1270–6.

13. Gottenberg JE, Guillevin L, Lambotte O et al. Tolerance and short term efficacy of rituximab in 43 patients with systemic autoimmune diseases. *Ann Rheum Dis* 2005;64:913–20.

14. Bowman SJ, Booth DA, Platts RG et al. Validation of a Sicca Symptoms Inventory for clinical studies of Sjögren's syndrome. *J Rheumatol* 2003;30:1259–66.

15. Pillemer SR, Smith J, Fox PC, Bowman SJ. Outcome measures for Sjögren's syndrome, April 10–11, 2003, Bethesda, Maryland, USA. *J Rheumatol* 2005;32:143–9.

16. Anaya JM, Rivera D, Palacio LG et al. D6S439 microsatellite identifies a new susceptibility region for primary Sjögren's syndrome. *J Rheumatol* 2003;30:2152–6.

17. Sordet C, Gottenberg JE, Goetz J et al. Anti-α-fodrin autoantibodies are not useful diagnostic markers of primary Sjögren's syndrome. *Ann Rheum Dis* 2005;64:1244–5.

18. Gordon TP, Cavill D, Neufing P et al. ICA69 autoantibodies in primary Sjögren's syndrome. *Lupus* 2004;13:483–4.

19. Dawson LJ, Allison HE, Stanbury J et al. Putative anti-muscarinic antibodies cannot be detected in patients with primary Sjögren's syndrome using conventional immunological approaches. *Rheumatology (Oxford)* 2004;43:1488–95.

20. Moyes DL, Martin A, Sawcer S et al. The distribution of the endogenous retroviruses HERV-K113 and HERV-K115 in health and disease. *Genomics* 2005;86:337–41.

21. Shim GJ, Warner M, Kim HJ et al. Aromatase-deficient mice spontaneously develop a lympho-proliferative autoimmune disease resembling Sjögren's syndrome. *Proc Natl Acad Sci USA* 2004;101: 12628–33

22. Barone F, Bombardieri M, Manzo A et al. Association of CXCL13 and CCL21 expression with the progressive organization of lymphoid-like structures in Sjögren's syndrome. *Arthritis Rheum* 2005;52:1773–84.

23. Hansen A, Reiter K, Ziprian T et al. Dysregulation of chemokine receptor expression and function by B cells of patients with primary Sjögren's syndrome. *Arthritis Rheum* 2005;52:2109–19.

24. Ogawa N, Kawanami T, Shimoyama K et al. Expression of interferon-inducible T cell alpha chemoattractant (CXCL11) in the salivary glands of patients with Sjögren's syndrome. *Clin Immunol* 2004;112:235–8.

25. Gottenberg JE, Busson M, Cohen-Solal J et al. Correlation of serum B lymphocyte stimulator and beta2 microglobulin with autoantibody secretion and systemic involvement in primary Sjögren's syndrome. *Ann Rheum Dis* 2005; 64:1050–5.

26. Jonsson MV, Szodoray P, Jellestad S et al. Association between circulating levels of the novel TNF family members APRIL and BAFF and lymphoid organization in primary Sjögren's syndrome. *J Clin Immunol* 2005;25:189–201.

27. Hjelmervik TO, Petersen K, Jonassen I et al. Gene expression profiling of minor salivary glands clearly distinguishes primary Sjögren's syndrome patients from healthy control subjects. *Arthritis Rheum* 2005;52:1534–44.

Ultrasound diagnosis of vasculitis

Wolfgang A Schmidt MD
Medical Center for Rheumatology Berlin–Buch, Berlin, Germany

Vasculitides may involve small vessels (e.g. Wegener's granulomatosis and most secondary vasculitides), medium-sized arteries (e.g. polyarteritis nodosa and Kawasaki's disease), or large arteries (temporal arteritis [giant-cell arteritis, GCA] and Takayasu's arteritis). In addition, 'large-vessel GCA' describes vasculitis of the distal subclavian, axillary and proximal brachial arteries.[1] It may occur with or without temporal artery vasculitis. Furthermore, the increased application of imaging techniques is revealing a growing number of patients with idiopathic aortitis (chronic periaortitis).[2]

In small-vessel vasculitides, ultrasound delineates secondary pathologies, but it is not capable of depicting pathognomonic findings.

Medium-sized artery vasculitides may cause aneurysms. In Kawasaki's disease, the detection of coronary artery aneurysms with either echocardiography or coronary angiography can establish the diagnosis if fever is present, according to the diagnostic guidelines of the American Heart Association.[3]

In large-vessel vasculitides, ultrasound delineates characteristic homogeneous wall swelling (Figure 1) and can be used to image the temporal, subclavian, carotid, axillary and other arteries. However, ultrasound cannot depict vessels that are localized behind bone or lungs, such as the proximal left subclavian artery and the thoracic descending aorta. Modern transducers provide resolutions of 0.1 mm.

In color Doppler ultrasound, the information on blood flow is integrated in the gray-scale image as a color signal. Duplex ultrasound is the combination of real-time imaging and Doppler ultrasound, enabling blood-flow characteristics, wall elasticity and plaques to be assessed.

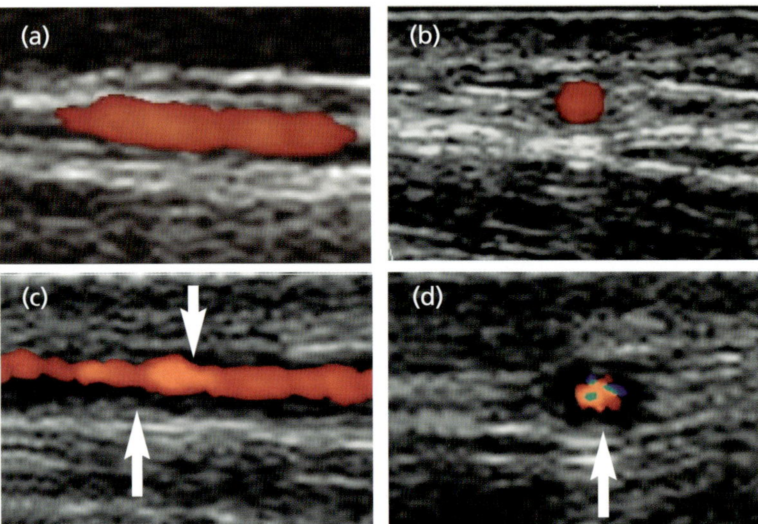

Figure 1 Color Doppler ultrasound image of temporal arteries. (a) Longitudinal and (b) transverse view of a normal frontal branch. (c) Longitudinal and (d) transverse view of edematous hypoechoic wall swelling (arrowed) of a parietal branch in a patient with active temporal arteritis.

In temporal arteritis

The ultrasound image of an inflamed temporal artery is characterized by three typical findings.[4,5]

- Edematous wall swelling: a dark, hypoechoic, circumferential wall thickening ('halo') appears around the lumen of the temporal artery (Figure 1). In most patients, it resolves within 2–3 weeks with corticosteroid treatment.
- Stenosis: narrowing of the vessel lumen leads to increased blood flow velocities and turbulences. Ultrasound shows a mixture of colors and persisting color signals in diastole. Doppler curves confirm this finding if the blood-flow velocity is more than twice the rate recorded in the area proximal to stenoses, perhaps with wave forms demonstrating turbulence and reduced velocity distal to stenoses.
- Occlusion: the image delineates a temporal artery with no color signals in it.

Equipment and experience. To perform accurate ultrasonography, one needs high-quality color Doppler ultrasound equipment, including a linear probe with a frequency above 8 MHz, experience in vascular ultrasonography, knowledge of the appearance of a normal temporal artery and standardized machine adjustments. The color signal should cover the entire artery lumen exactly. If it extends over parts of the vessel wall, minor wall edema may be missed. On the other hand, if the color signal only covers the center of the lumen, false hypoechoic areas may appear. Anechogenicity represents fluid, while hypoechogenicity represents edematous tissue. The color sample steering should have an angle of 20–30 degrees. The sonographer should have studied at least 50 people with normal temporal arteries before attempting to diagnose temporal arteritis. The superficial temporal artery with the parietal and longitudinal branch should be investigated in two planes on both sides in full length.

Sensitivity and specificity. A meta-analysis of duplex ultrasound in 23 studies involving 2036 subjects described sensitivity of 87% and specificity of 96% in terms of the clinical diagnosis.[6] Pretest probabilities of GCA of 10%, 50% and 90% increased to 71%, 96% and 99%, respectively, after positive findings with duplex ultrasound. They decreased to 2%, 12% and 55%, respectively, with negative ultrasound findings. The sensitivities and specificities were comparable with temporal artery histology.

Ultrasound versus biopsy. Temporal artery histology is still the gold standard for diagnosis, though it has disadvantages, including its invasiveness, the length of time it takes to obtain a result, and the false-negative results obtained in some patients because of skip lesions. Ultrasound carried out by an experienced sonographer (with proven high specificities for the diagnosis of temporal arteritis) may replace biopsy. In our center, where we have performed 1500 ultrasound examinations and have had 180 newly diagnosed patients with active GCA in the last 12 years, we perform biopsy only in ambiguous cases. In a person with typical clinical signs and a 'halo', we rely on the ultrasound results, as the specificity is 99.5% in our series. However, if we detect only stenoses (specificity 96%), we perform biopsy.

Gadolinium-enhanced magnetic resonance imaging (MRI). Recent studies with gadolinium-enhanced MRI have produced similar images of the temporal and occipital arteries. Sensitivities and specificities for the diagnosis of GCA are comparable with duplex ultrasound.[7]

In polymyalgia rheumatica

In one study, temporal artery ultrasound in patients with polymyalgia rheumatica (PMR) assisted with the diagnosis of temporal arteritis in 7 of 102 patients with 'pure' PMR.[8] In another, ultrasound of the shoulder was shown to typically detect small amounts of fluid in the subdeltoid bursa and around the long biceps tendon. Minor effusions of the glenohumeral joint were also common.[9] In addition, ultrasound has often been helpful in the detection of trochanteric bursitis and hip joint synovitis.[10]

In large-vessel giant-cell arteritis

The axillary arteries are easily accessible by ultrasound. Duplex axillary artery ultrasound aids diagnosis in patients with suspected GCA or PMR, when performed in addition to clinical assessment with auscultation of the axillary region, palpation of radial pulses and bilateral measurement of blood pressure. The wall swelling is hypoechoic in untreated active disease, as described in the temporal arteries. It frequently persists at follow-up, but it becomes brighter with treatment because of fibrosis. In patients with GCA, wall edema may occur in other arteries, such as the carotid, facial, occipital, vertebral, subclavian, radial, ulnar and popliteal arteries. Up to 40% of patients with GCA may exhibit vasculitis of the axillary arteries, depicted by ultrasound or positron emission tomography (PET).[11] A 100% correlation has been described between ultrasound and PET in the detection of large-vessel GCA.[12]

Highlights in ultrasound diagnosis of vasculitis *2005–06*

WHAT'S IN?

- Meta-analysis of results from duplex ultrasound of temporal arteries
- Diagnosis of temporal arteritis based on typical clinical signs and an ultrasound examination that clearly demonstrates edematous wall swelling
- Temporal artery biopsy for ambiguous cases
- The use of ultrasound to reveal subdeltoid bursitis, biceps tenosynovitis, trochanteric bursitis and hip joint synovitis in polymyalgia rheumatica (PMR)

WHAT'S OUT?

- Concentrating only on clinical findings at the temporal arteries. In patients with giant-cell arteritis (GCA) and PMR, auscultation of the axillary region should be performed and the pulse status of the patient assessed; ultrasound frequently detects vasculitis of axillary arteries in patients with GCA

In Takayasu's arteritis

Takayasu's arteritis occurs predominantly in young women. The subclavian arteries are most commonly involved (93%), followed by the aorta (65%) and the common carotid arteries (58%). Vasculitis of other arteries is common. Ultrasound reveals characteristic long segments of smooth, homogeneous, midechoic, concentric wall thickening. It is, in general, brighter than in temporal arteritis and large-vessel GCA, which is consistent with the more chronic course of the condition, with less vessel wall edema.[13] Arteriosclerotic lesions are inhomogeneous and irregular, with calcifications.

In other vasculitides

Small-vessel vasculitides such as Wegener's granulomatosis sometimes involve temporal arteries[14] or finger arteries.[15] Ultrasound of finger arteries displays occlusion but no wall swelling. The ultrasound image of temporal vasculitis cannot differentiate between GCA and other forms of vasculitis. Therefore, one should look for other systemic vasculitides if biopsy is not performed, by assessing the patient for antineutrophil cytoplasmic antibodies (ANCA), proteinuria, pulmonary infiltrates or nodules and nasal sinus infiltrates.[16]

References

1. Matteson EL. Large vessel involvement in giant cell arteritis: incidence, predictors, and mortality. *Rheumatology* 2005;44(suppl 3): 10–11.

2. Jois RN, Gaffney K, Marshall T et al. Chronic periaortitis – a missed rheumatological disease. *Rheumatology* 2005;44(suppl 3):19.

3. Newburger JW, Takahashi M, Gerber MA et al. Diagnosis, treatment, and long-term management of Kawasaki disease: a statement for health professionals from the Committee on Rheumatic Fever, Endocarditis, and Kawasaki Disease, Council on Cardiovascular Disease in the Young, American Heart Association. *Pediatrics* 2004;114:1708–33.

4. Schmidt WA, Kraft HE, Vorpahl K et al. Color duplex ultrasonography in the diagnosis of temporal arteritis. *N Engl J Med* 1997;337:1336–42.

5. Schmidt WA. Doppler sonography in rheumatology. *Best Pract Res Clin Rheumatol* 2004;18:827–46.

6. Karassa FB, Matsagas MI, Schmidt WA, Ioannidis JP. Meta-analysis: test performance of ultrasonography for giant-cell arteritis. *Ann Intern Med* 2005;142:359–69.

7. Bley TA, Wieben O, Uhl M et al. High-resolution MRI in giant cell arteritis: imaging of the wall of the superficial temporal artery. *Am J Roentgenol* 2005;184:283–7.

8. Schmidt WA, Gromnica-Ihle E. Incidence of temporal arteritis in patients with polymyalgia rheumatica: a prospective study using colour Doppler ultrasonography of the temporal arteries. *Rheumatology (Oxford)* 2002;41:46–52.

9. Cantini F, Salvarani C, Olivieri I et al. Shoulder ultrasonography in the diagnosis of polymyalgia rheumatica: a case-control study. *J Rheumatol* 2001;28:1049–55.

10. Cantini F, Niccoli L, Nannini C et al. Inflammatory changes of hip synovial structures in polymyalgia rheumatica. *Clin Exp Rheumatol* 2005;23:462–8.

11. Schmidt WA, Blockmans D. Use of ultrasonography and positron emission tomography in the diagnosis and assessment of large-vessel vasculitis. *Curr Opin Rheumatol* 2005,17:9–15.

12. Brodmann M, Lipp RW, Passath A et al. The role of 2-18F-fluoro-2-deoxy-D-glucose positron emission tomography in the diagnosis of giant cell arteritis of the temporal arteries. *Rheumatology (Oxford)* 2004;43:241–2.

13. Ringleb PA, Strittmatter EI, Loewer M et al. Cerebrovascular manifestations of Takayasu arteritis in Europe. *Rheumatology (Oxford)* 2005;44:1012–15.

14. Müller E, Schneider W, Kettritz U et al. Temporal arteritis with pauci-immune glomerulonephritis: a systemic disease. *Clin Nephrol* 2004;62:384–6.

15. Schmidt WA, Wernicke D, Kiefer E, Gromnica-Ihle E. Colour duplex sonography of finger arteries in vasculitis and in systemic sclerosis. *Ann Rheum Dis* 2006;65:265–7.

16. Schmidt WA, Gromnica-Ihle E. What is the best approach to diagnose large-vessel vasculitis? *Best Pract Res Clin Rheumatol* 2005;19:223–42.

Hematopoietic stem-cell transplantation

Jacob M van Laar* MD and Alan Tyndall† MD
*Department of Rheumatology, Leiden University Medical Center, The Netherlands; †Department of Rheumatology, University Hospital, Basel, Switzerland

Hematopoietic stem-cell transplantation (HSCT) is the short name for a technically complex treatment aimed at resetting the dysregulated immune system of patients suffering from severe autoimmune disease. It was introduced to the arena of clinical rheumatology in the mid-1990s after observations of remission of autoimmune disease in experimental animal models and in patients treated with HSCT for hematologic malignancies.[1]

HSCT differs from therapies that modulate a single cell type (e.g. B-cell-depleting antibodies) or cytokine (tumor necrosis factor [TNF] inhibitors) in that it targets a wide array of immune-competent cells, including B and T cells, thus creating space for the generation of a new immunologic repertoire from hematopoietic stem cells. Compared with conventional immunosuppressive drugs, HSCT has a more fundamental effect on the acquired immune system, in effect 'resetting' it.[2]

Harvesting hematopoietic stem cells

Hematopoietic stem cells (HSC) (i.e. the progenitor cells of red blood cells, platelets and all lineages of the immune system) reside in the bone marrow, but can be driven into the blood by a procedure called mobilization. This is achieved by administering one or two bolus infusions of cyclophosphamide followed by subcutaneous injections with granulocyte-colony stimulating factor. These cells are then isolated from blood by leukapheresis, a procedure in which blood is drained via a venous catheter to a blood-cell separation device. After the white blood cells, including stem cells, have been removed, all other components of the blood are returned to the circulation via another venous catheter. The white cell collection (known as the 'graft product') is subsequently processed in the laboratory to obtain an enriched stem-cell fraction, which is cryopreserved until later use at transplantation.

HSCs can be procured from:

- the patient's own blood or bone marrow – autologous
- a monozygotic twin – syngeneic
- a non-identical donor – allogeneic.

Allogeneic transplantation has become less acutely toxic as non-myeloablative conditioning regimens (misleadingly referred to as 'mini-transplantation') have been introduced. However, the fact that the risk of graft-versus-host disease (leading to significant morbidity) remains unchanged, together with the limited availability of matched donors (siblings), puts constraints on the wider application of this modality. Autologous HSCT has therefore been most commonly employed in the context of autoimmune disease.

Transplantation

The main therapeutic component of HSCT routinely takes place several weeks after stem-cell harvest. The transplant recipient receives high-dose chemotherapy with or without cytotoxic antibodies, or total body irradiation, to eradicate the existing immune cells; granulocytes, red blood cells and platelets are also affected. To minimize the risks of infection or bleeding, the graft product is re-infused (also named 'transplantation'). The infused stem cells give rise to new immune cells that replace the original 'sick' immune cells. This process is, in part, stochastic (i.e. determined by chance). The basic steps of harvest and transplantation are summarized in Figure 1.

Risks. HSCT is an intensive treatment with risks of severe, sometimes fatal, complications, including infections, bleeding, heart failure, respiratory insufficiency, renal failure and lymphoma. Less severe but more frequent (and usually reversible) toxicities include nausea, fever, alopecia, infertility, arthralgia, myalgia and menstrual disorders. The patient is usually hospitalized for several weeks while

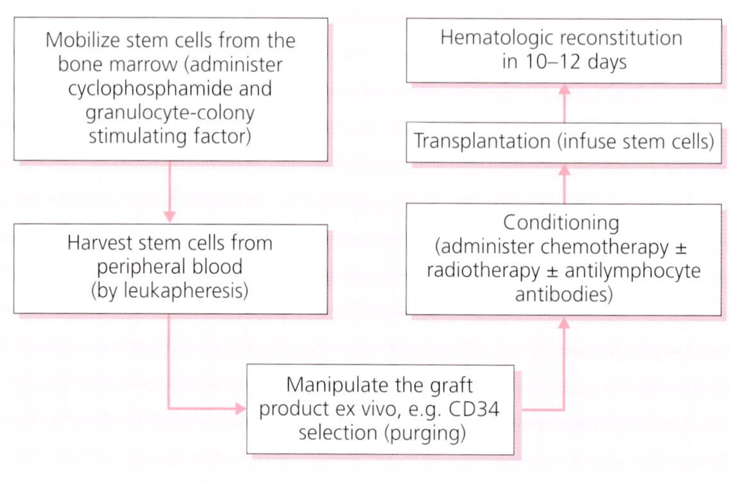

Figure 1 Steps in autologous, peripheral blood hematopoietic stem-cell transplantation.

the procedure is performed, and afterwards to cover any unwanted consequences of the therapy. Antibiotic treatment and transfusions of red blood cells or platelets are usually necessary in the period immediately following the transplantation.

HSCT would not have been considered as a treatment option in autoimmune disease had it not been recognized that severe autoimmune diseases are associated with excess morbidity and early mortality. The lifespan of patients with severe rheumatoid arthritis (RA) is approximately 7 years less than normal, and 10-year survival of patients with severe systemic sclerosis or refractory lupus erythematosus can be as low as 50–80%. In these patients, HSCT may be justified.

Clinical experience in rheumatic autoimmune disease

Based on experiences in Europe, where over 200 patients with rheumatic diseases received HSCT between 1995 and 2005, the feasibility of the procedure in autoimmune disease has now been firmly established. Trends regarding safety and efficacy have emerged from registry analyses and pilot studies.[3] More intense regimens were associated with higher treatment-related mortality but a lower probability of relapse, though differences in regimens, patient entry criteria and outcome parameters preclude more refined analyses.

Safety. Importantly, the safety of HSCT has improved, as illustrated by the marked decrease in transplant-related mortality (TRM) in patients with severe systemic sclerosis (SSc): TRM dropped from 17% in the first cohort of 41 patients entered in a European database, to 8.7% in a more recent analysis of 65 patients (which included the original 41 patients),[4] to 0% in the 29 patients randomized so far to the transplant arm of the Autologous Stem cell Transplantation International Scleroderma (ASTIS) trial (discussed below).

With few exceptions, there have been no reports of unexpected toxicities such as lymphomas or opportunistic infections beyond those known to be associated with HSCT in general. Major adverse events have been documented though, most notably in SSc, systemic lupus erythematosus (SLE) and juvenile idiopathic arthritis (JIA).[5,6] These included respiratory insufficiency during conditioning (in SSc), graft failure (in SLE) and macrophage-activation syndrome (in JIA), and accounted for the majority of TRM in these diseases. These problems have become manageable with modifications of protocols (e.g. by less intense T-cell depletion in JIA, and by lung shielding during total body irradiation in SSc), and by excluding patients with advanced disease.

Efficacy. Once feasibility and safety had been established, attention turned to efficacy, as impressive clinical responses were being observed. Striking differences in responsiveness and toxicity were noted, depending on the disease targeted (Figure 2), though differences in protocols may have acted as potential confounders.

In juvenile idiopathic arthritis. The majority of patients with JIA experienced marked improvements in disease activity, functional ability and quality of life, with growth restored after

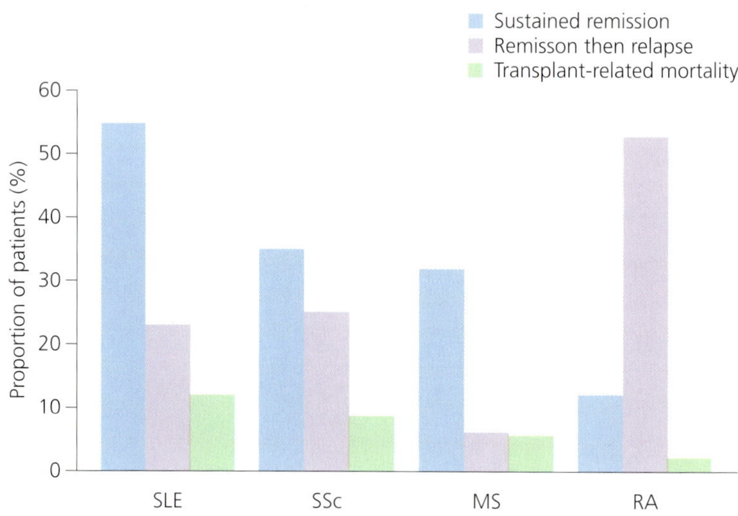

Figure 2 Selected outcomes of sustained remission, remission then relapse and treatment-related mortality after hematopoietic stem-cell transplantation in patients with four different autoimmune diseases: SLE, systemic lupus erythematosus (n = 53); SSc, systemic sclerosis (n = 57); MS, multiple sclerosis (n = 85); RA, rheumatoid arthritis (n = 73).

the discontinuation of corticosteroid therapy.[6] In many children, immunosuppression ceased for several years after HSCT, though late relapses have occurred.

In systemic sclerosis. Of those patients with established generalized skin thickening, the majority who received HSCT experienced durable skin softening, defying conventional wisdom that fibrotic skin abnormalities are irreversible.[4]

In systemic lupus erythematosus disease activity, as measured by the SLE disease activity index (SLEDAI), improved dramatically, and lung function tests in patients with pulmonary abnormalities indicated significant improvements.[5,7]

In rheumatoid arthritis. Most patients with RA showed only transient responses, as measured by scores of disease activity, functional ability, quality of life and rate of joint destruction. However, the disease appeared to be more amenable to conventional antirheumatic medications after stem-cell transplantation.[8,9]

Interestingly, two syngeneic HSCTs in patients with RA have been reported, one with a long-lasting remission,[10] the other with a rapid relapse;[11] an allogeneic HSCT in another patient also resulted in remission of RA.[12]

Prospective controlled trials

Building on experience from pilot studies, initiatives were taken in Europe and the USA to further investigate the therapeutic value of HSCT in autoimmune disease through prospective, multicenter trials.

The first of these, the ASTIS trial, was launched in 2001 under the auspices of the European Group for Blood and Marrow Transplantation (EBMT) and the European League Against Rheumatism (EULAR) to compare the safety and efficacy of HSCT with that of conventional pulse-therapy cyclophosphamide in patients with severe SSc at risk of early mortality.[13] At the time of publication (March 2006), 65 patients from 20 European centers have been randomized to either the HSCT or control arms. No unexpected toxicities or treatment-related mortality have been observed so far, but long-term follow-up of patients is crucial in order to monitor potential late sequelae or to discover delayed diverging trends in (event-free) survival.

Similar randomized trials have started or are being planned for patients with severe SLE, multiple sclerosis (MS) and Crohn's disease.

Mechanistic aspects

The profound degree of immunosuppression attained with HSCT has generated interesting data on the mechanistic aspects of this treatment. Researchers have found that specific autoantibodies do not disappear after HSCT, despite long-term remissions. This has been consistently observed for Scl-70 autoantibodies in patients with scleroderma, indicating that these autoantibodies were produced by non-dividing long-lived plasma cells. Titers of rheumatoid factors dropped in patients with RA after HSCT, but failed to normalize.

They returned to pretreatment levels before relapse, in keeping with data from patients with RA treated with rituximab. In many patients with SLE, antinuclear antibodies and anti-double-stranded-DNA antibodies disappeared after HSCT, but returned to detectable levels during relapse.

HSCT has been shown not only to affect B-cell populations, but also to perturb profoundly the T-cell compartment, as illustrated by the normalization of the dysregulated T-cell receptor repertoires in patients with MS and SLE.[14] In patients with JIA, the numbers of functionally active $CD4^{+}$ $CD25^{+}$ regulatory T cells increased after HSCT, evidence that HSCT restores immunoregulatory mechanisms.[15] In patients with RA, analyses of lymphocytes infiltrating synovial tissue suggest that relapse originates from lesional T cells that were not eliminated by immunoablation.[16]

Highlights in **hematopoietic stem-cell transplantation** *2005–06*

WHAT'S IN?

- Randomized clinical trials of autologous hematopoietic stem-cell transplantation (HSCT) in patients with refractory autoimmune diseases
- Careful selection of potential subjects to avoid complications after HSCT
- Investigation for potential biomarkers of immune modulation after HSCT

WHAT'S OUT?

- Autologous HSCT in unselected patients with refractory autoimmune diseases outside formal clinical trials
- The use of autologous HSCT in patients with rheumatoid arthritis for whom the benefits are transient

References

1. van Bekkum DW. Stem cell transplantation for autoimmune disorders. Preclinical experiments. *Best Pract Res Clin Haematol* 2004;17:201–22.

2. van Laar JM, Tyndall A. Intense immunosuppression and stem-cell transplantation for patients with severe rheumatic autoimmune disease: a review. *Cancer Control* 2003;10:57–65.

3. Gratwohl A, Passweg J, Bocelli-Tyndall C et al. Autologous hematopoietic stem cell transplantation for autoimmune diseases. *Bone Marrow Transplant* 2005;35:869–79.

4. Farge D, Passweg J, van Laar JM et al. Autologous stem cell transplantation in the treatment of systemic sclerosis: report from the EBMT/EULAR Registry. *Ann Rheum Dis* 2004;63:974–81.

5. Jayne D, Passweg J, Marmont A et al. Autologous stem cell transplantation for systemic lupus erythematosus. *Lupus* 2004;13:168–76.

6. De Kleer IM, Brinkman DM, Ferster A et al. Autologous stem cell transplantation for refractory juvenile idiopathic arthritis: analysis of clinical effects, mortality, and transplant related morbidity. *Ann Rheum Dis* 2004;63:1318–26.

7. Traynor AE, Corbridge TC, Eagan AE et al. Prevalence and reversibility of pulmonary dysfunction in refractory systemic lupus: improvement correlates with disease remission following hematopoietic stem cell transplantation. *Chest* 2005;127:1680–9.

8. Teng YK, Verburg RJ, Sont JK et al. Long-term follow up of health status in patients with severe rheumatoid arthritis after high-dose chemotherapy followed by autologous hematopoietic stem cell transplantation. *Arthritis Rheum* 2005;52:2272–6.

9. Snowden JA, Passweg J, Moore JJ et al. Autologous hemopoietic stem cell transplantation in severe rheumatoid arthritis: a report from the EBMT and ABMTR. *J Rheumatol* 2004;31:482–8.

10. McColl GJ, Szer J, Wicks IP. Sustained remission, possibly cure, of seronegative arthritis after high-dose chemotherapy and syngeneic hematopoietic stem cell transplantation. *Arthritis Rheum* 2005;52:3322.

11. van Oosterhout MR, Verburg RJ, Levarht EW et al. High dose chemotherapy and syngeneic stem cell transplantation in a patient with refractory rheumatoid arthritis: poor response associated with persistence of host autoantibodies and synovial abnormalities. *Ann Rheum Dis* 2005; 64:1783–5.

12. Burt RK, Oyama Y, Verda L et al. Induction of remission of severe and refractory rheumatoid arthritis by allogeneic mixed chimerism. *Arthritis Rheum* 2004;50:2466–70.

13. van Laar JM, Farge D, Tyndall A. Autologous Stem cell Transplantation International Scleroderma (ASTIS) trial: hope on the horizon for patients with severe systemic sclerosis. *Ann Rheum Dis* 2005;64:1515.

14. Muraro PA, Douek DC, Packer A et al. Thymic output generates a new and diverse TCR repertoire after autologous stem cell transplantation in multiple sclerosis patients. *J Exp Med* 2005;201:805–16.

15. de Kleer I, Vastert B, Klein M et al. Autologous stem cell transplantation for autoimmunity induces immunologic self-tolerance by reprogramming autoreactive T-cells and restoring the CD4+CD25+ immune regulatory network. *Blood* 2006;107:1696–702.

16. Verburg RJ, Flierman R, Sont JK et al. Outcome of intensive immunosuppression and autologous stem cell transplantation in patients with severe rheumatoid arthritis is associated with the composition of synovial T cell infiltration. *Ann Rheum Dis* 2005;64:1397–405.

Therapeutic tissue engineering

Anthony P Hollander BSc, PhD
Academic Rheumatology, University of Bristol, UK

The use of cells to regenerate tissues offers a new paradigm in the treatment of musculoskeletal disorders. Cell therapy for cartilage repair is already well established, while potentially important methods for engineering bone tissue are now being developed.

Autologous chondrocyte implantation

Autologous chondrocyte implantation (ACI) was developed by Peterson and colleagues more than 15 years ago, as a method for the repair of focal cartilage lesions.[1,2] The technique involved taking a small biopsy of low-weight-bearing cartilage from the injured knee, isolating the chondrocytes enzymatically, expanding them under sterile conditions and then injecting the expanded population into the debrided lesion beneath a flap of periosteal tissue. Implantation of the flap requires extensive suturing and cannot be performed arthroscopically.

Early results were clinically promising, and subsequent follow-up studies have demonstrated significant improvement for selected patient groups over 9 years.[3] However, problems with hypertrophy of the periosteal flap led to the adoption of a porcine collagen I/III membrane to cover the lesion, which significantly reduced this side effect, although the flap still required suturing in place.[4] A recent randomized trial comparing ACI with an alternative cartilage repair technique known as microfracture revealed no significant difference between them, with both approaches producing acceptable short-term clinical results.[5] A separate retrospective analysis comparing ACI with mosaicplasty (autologous transplantation of osteochondral plugs) found that average costs were higher for ACI and there was no significant difference in clinical outcome, although ACI-treated patients tended to fare better.[6] Mosaicplasty, however, requires the removal of numerous large osteochondral plugs from the low-weight-bearing cartilage of the knee and the consequences for these donor sites are not well understood.[7]

Cells seeded onto membranes

A variant of ACI involves seeding the chondrocytes onto a membrane, which can then be implanted with or without fibrin glue. This approach has the advantage of being suture free and therefore it can be provided arthroscopically. Two membrane-assisted technologies have emerged in clinical practice. The matrix-associated ACI (MACI) technique (Verigen, Germany) utilizes a collagen I/III bilayer membrane. A recent study compared MACI with ACI and found no significant difference in outcome.[4] The authors concluded that although the technical advantages of handling the MACI implant are attractive, longer-term studies are needed before the technique can be widely adopted. The second technique, Hyalograft®C (Fidia Advanced Biopolymers, Italy), uses a biodegradable esterified hyaluronic acid membrane. Three recent clinical studies have shown efficacy equivalent to that of ACI,[8–10] and analysis of biopsies from patients treated with this technique have demonstrated excellent restoration of hyaline cartilage structure in approximately 50% of cases.[11,12] Interestingly, cartilage repair was not inhibited in patients with early osteoarthritis noted on X-ray at the time of implantation, and the regenerative process may even have been enhanced in this group.[12]

Gene therapy

A variant approach to cell therapy is the use of genes to promote specific cellular responses. Gene therapy could be achieved by transducing chondrocytes while they are being cultured in the laboratory and then transferring them into patients.[13] This approach would be particularly attractive for eliciting localized cartilage effects without risking systemic expression of the transgene; potentially it could be used to treat patients with advanced osteoarthritis in whom cells alone might not provide enough regenerative capacity.

Another approach is to use synovial fibroblasts to carry the transgene into the joint. This is less invasive because no surgical implantation is required, only intra-articular injection. Therefore, the technique can be used for small joints as well as large ones. This localized delivery of genes into joints is a particularly attractive concept for patients with rheumatoid arthritis (RA). An exciting phase I clinical study has now demonstrated that a retroviral interleukin-1 receptor antagonist gene can be safely delivered into the metacarpophalangeal joints of patients with advanced RA.[14] This is a major step forward and offers the real prospect of an effective gene therapy protocol.

Tissue engineering in vivo

The cartilage repair techniques highlighted above have been established for the treatment of relatively small, focal defects. Treatment of larger defects of cartilage as well as bone will require growth of large implants. To achieve this in vitro is technically very challenging and would require a sophisticated bioreactor. An alternative approach would be to engineer the tissue in vivo, within the patient's own body. An important new study has described just such an approach.[15] The in-vivo bioreactor was developed primarily for the production of large pieces of bone, but under appropriate conditions it can be adapted for the formation of cartilage. The bone that is formed is of high quality and is thought by the authors to have particular application in spinal fusion procedures. Furthermore, the approach could be used to generate bone for banking and subsequent transplantation.

Stem cells

There is growing interest in the use of stem cells to generate cells of a specific lineage for tissue engineering therapies. A recent review of mesenchymal stem cells gives a good description of the potential use of a patient's own bone-marrow stromal population for musculoskeletal cell therapies and the use of 'cell painting' to target

Highlights in **therapeutic tissue engineering** *2005–06*

WHAT'S IN?

- Collagen and hyaluronic acid membranes to assist autologous chondrocyte implantation
- Growing tissues in vivo
- Gene therapy for rheumatoid arthritis
- Stem-cell therapy

WHAT'S OUT?

- Use of a periosteal flap in autologous chondrocyte implantation

these cells to specific sites in the body.[16] It is uncertain whether human bone marrow contains truly primitive stem cells rather than committed progenitors. However, a study of nucleostemin, which has been described as a stem-cell marker, has demonstrated the presence of significant numbers of more primitive stem cells in adult bone marrow, suggesting that the mesenchymal population is not just made up of progenitors.[17]

There is also a growing interest in the potential of human embryonic stem-cell (hES) therapy, as described in a number of reviews.[18–20] One of the problems of utilizing hES is that they are generally thought to have to form embryoid bodies in vitro before differentiating, which limits the rate at which specifically differentiated cells can be generated. However, a new study has demonstrated that one particular hES line (H9) is capable of forming osteogenic cells without the need for embryoid body formation.[21] This observation suggests that therapeutic use of hES may be feasible. Another study has suggested that chondrocytes can be generated from hES, though in that case embryoid body formation was required.[22]

References

1. Peterson L. Articular cartilage injuries treated with autologous chondrocyte transplantation in the human knee. *Acta Orthop Belg* 1996;62(suppl 1):196–200.

2. Brittberg M, Lindahl A, Nilsson A et al. Treatment of deep cartilage defects in the knee with autologous chondrocyte transplantation. *N Engl J Med* 1994;331:889–95.

3. Peterson L, Minas T, Brittberg M et al. Two- to 9-year outcome after autologous chondrocyte transplantation of the knee. *Clin Orthop Relat Res* 2000;374:212–34.

4. Bartlett W, Skinner JA, Gooding CR et al. Autologous chondrocyte implantation versus matrix-induced autologous chondrocyte implantation for osteochondral defects of the knee: a prospective, randomised study. *J Bone Joint Surg Br* 2005;87:640–5.

5. Knutsen G, Engebretsen L, Ludvigsen TC et al. Autologous chondrocyte implantation compared with microfracture in the knee. A randomized trial. *J Bone Joint Surg Am* 2004;86-A:455–64.

6. Derrett S, Stokes EA, James M et al. Cost and health status analysis after autologous chondrocyte implantation and mosaicplasty: a retrospective comparison. *Int J Technol Assess Health Care* 2005;21:359–67.

7. Hangody L, Feczko P, Bartha L et al. Mosaicplasty for the treatment of articular defects of the knee and ankle. *Clin Orthop Relat Res* 2001;391(suppl):S328–36.

8. Marcacci M, Berruto M, Brocchetta D et al. Articular cartilage engineering with Hyalograft C: 3-year clinical results. *Clin Orthop Relat Res* 2005;435:96–105.

9. Trattnig S, Ba-Ssalamah A, Pinker K et al. Matrix-based autologous chondrocyte implantation for cartilage repair: noninvasive monitoring by high-resolution magnetic resonance imaging. *Magn Reson Imaging* 2005;23:779–87.

10. Nehrer S, Domayer S, Dorotka R et al. Three-year clinical outcome after chondrocyte transplantation using a hyaluronan matrix for cartilage repair. *Eur J Radiol* 2006;57:3–8.

11. Dickinson SC, Sims TJ, Pittarello L et al. Quantitative outcome measures of cartilage repair in patients treated by tissue engineering. *Tissue Eng* 2005;11:277–87.

12. Hollander AP, Dickinson SC, Sims TJ et al. Maturation of engineered cartilage implanted in injured and osteoarthritic human knees. *Tissue Eng* 2006; in press.

13. Kafienah W, Al-Fayez F, Hollander AP, Barker MD. Inhibition of cartilage degradation: a combined tissue engineering and gene therapy approach. *Arthritis Rheum* 2003;48:709–18.

14. Evans CH, Robbins PD, Ghivizzani SC et al. Gene transfer to human joints: progress toward a gene therapy of arthritis. *Proc Natl Acad Sci USA* 2005;102:8698–703.

15. Stevens MM, Marini RP, Schaefer D et al. In vivo engineering of organs: the bone bioreactor. *Proc Natl Acad Sci USA* 2005;102: 11450–5.

16. Caplan AI. Review: mesenchymal stem cells: cell-based reconstructive therapy in orthopedics. *Tissue Eng* 2005;11:1198–211.

17. Kafienah W, Mistry S, Williams C, Hollander AP. Nucleostemin is a marker of proliferating stromal stem cells in adult human bone marrow. *Stem Cells* 2005; Nov 10 [Epub ahead of print].

18. Mayhall EA, Paffett-Lugassy N, Zon LI. The clinical potential of stem cells. *Curr Opin Cell Biol* 2004;16: 713–20.

19. Gerecht-Nir S, Itskovitz-Eldor J. Cell therapy using human embryonic stem cells. *Transpl Immunol* 2004; 12:203–9.

20. Vats A, Bielby RC, Tolley NS et al. Stem cells. *Lancet* 2005; 366:592–602.

21. Karp JM, Ferreira LS, Khademhosseini A et al. Cultivation of human embryonic stem cells without the embryoid body step enhances osteogenesis in vitro. *Stem Cells* 2005; Nov 10 [Epub ahead of print].

22. Vats A, Bielby RC, Tolley N et al. Chondrogenic differentiation of human embryonic stem cells: the effect of the micro-environment. *Tissue Eng* 2006; in press.

Catastrophic antiphospholipid (Asherson's) syndrome

Ronald A Asherson MD FRCP FACP FCP FACR
Division of Immunology, School of Pathology, University of the Witwatersrand, Johannesburg, South Africa

Antiphospholipid syndrome (APS) has five known variants.

- Simple or 'classic' APS comprising predominantly large-vessel (venous and arterial) occlusions with minimal small-vessel occlusive disease (renal, retinal, skin etc.), as originally defined.[1]
- Catastrophic APS (CAPS; or Asherson's syndrome) with major small-vessel occlusive disease and minor large-vessel involvement.[2]
- Microangiopathic APS (MAPS), which comprises patients with thrombotic thrombocytopenic purpura (TTP)-like syndromes, HELLP syndrome, and heparin-induced thrombocytopenia (HIT) with circulating antiphospholipid antibodies (aPLs).[3] (The acronym HELLP derives from H, hemolysis; EL, elevated liver enzymes; LP, low blood level of platelets.)
- 'Seronegative' APS, which has essentially the same clinical features as simple APS but with persistently negative serology for aPL.[4]
- Systemic APS (Hughes' syndrome), which is essentially simple APS with systemic manifestations (e.g. valve lesions, adrenal failure, livedo reticularis, chorea).[5]

CAPS is a rapidly progressive variant of antiphospholipid syndrome.[6] It was first defined in 1992 with the publication of ten representative cases.[7] More than 300 cases have now been collected and most have been included on the website www.med.ub.es/MIMMUN/FORUM/CAPS.HTM. In 2003, the eponym Asherson's syndrome was attached.[1] The relationship of CAPS to APS is illustrated in Figure 1.

Most cases of CAPS are preceded by a primary or secondary APS (usually secondary to systemic lupus erythematosus [SLE] or 'lupus-like' disease). Following recovery from CAPS, 26% of

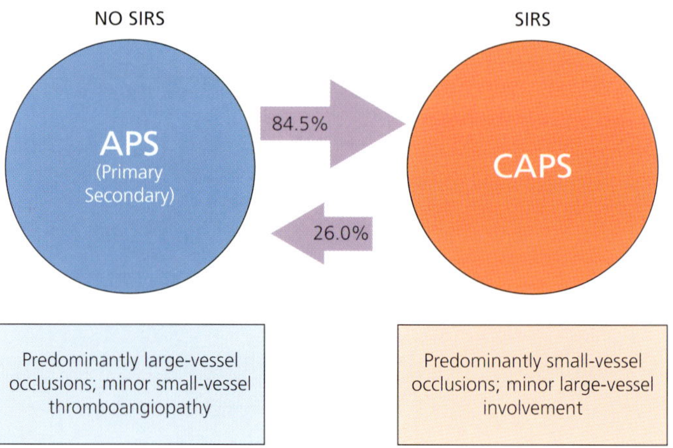

Figure 1 The relationship of catastrophic antiphospholipid syndrome (CAPS) to antiphospholipid syndrome (APS), showing that 84.5% of patients with CAPS have a history of 'primary' or 'secondary' APS, and that 26% of CAPS survivors may develop APS-related events in the future. SIRS, systemic inflammatory response syndrome.

patients may suffer recurrent simple APS manifestations (e.g. single thrombotic occlusions).

Clinical features

The characteristic clinical features of CAPS are:

- predominantly small-vessel occlusive disease resulting in multiple organ dysfunction syndrome (MODS)
- fulminant tissue necrosis, particularly involving the gastrointestinal tract, which may result in progressive features of the systemic inflammatory response syndrome (SIRS), often manifesting as an acute respiratory distress syndrome (ARDS)[8]
- a high frequency of unusual organ involvement (e.g. reproductive organ infarctions, bone-marrow necrosis, acalculous cholecystitis, polyneuropathy or splenic, hepatic and adrenal infarctions)
- serological evidence of disseminated intravascular coagulation (DIC) in a significant proportion of patients.[9]

Most patients end up in intensive care units with a plethora of physicians in attendance. It seems that the diagnosis is often missed by attending physicians at an early stage. This warrants an aggressive educational effort, as prompt and appropriately chosen therapies may be lifesaving.

The condition is most frequently encountered in patients with a 'primary' APS (PAPS) (49.9%), with the frequency in patients with SLE and 'lupus-like' disease being slightly lower (45%). Other less common associations include rheumatoid arthritis, systemic sclerosis, dermatomyositis, Crohn's disease, ulcerative colitis, polychondritis and some vasculitides (e.g. Behçet's syndrome).

As some patients may have already been identified as suffering from an APS and/or SLE, they may already be on long-term corticosteroids and/or anticoagulation therapy. The condition may arise de novo in others. A previous history of vascular occlusive events is therefore of major importance to physicians who suspect the diagnosis.

Triggering and precipitating factors

Triggering factors can be identified in 60% of patients as follows:

- infections (22%)
- trauma (13%)
- anticoagulation withdrawal (7%)
- neoplasia (7%)
- obstetric related (4%)
- lupus 'flares' (3%)
- drugs (captopril, oral contraceptives, danazol, thiazide diuretics), ovulation induction and postimmunization (4%).

Specific infections (e.g. typhoid, malaria and dengue fever) have been incriminated. In the majority of cases, a variety of non-specific infectious triggers have been reported; these include viral upper respiratory infections, unidentified bacterial urinary tract or gastrointestinal infections, and infected leg ulcers. Immunization against yellow fever, Japanese B encephalitis and influenza has been followed by CAPS in isolated cases.

Major or minor surgery (e.g. biopsy) may be a precipitating trauma, as may simple fractures. In some patients (approximately 5–10%), 'multiple' trigger factors are present within the same patient (e.g. infection, anticoagulation withdrawal followed by a surgical procedure or biopsy in patients with neoplasia who have aPL) – the so-called double- or treble-hit hypothesis, which is common to patients presenting with multiple organ failure from other causes (e.g. sepsis, burns, pancreatitis).

Predominantly, the kidneys (70%), lungs (66%), brain (60%), heart (52%) and skin (47%) are involved. Cardiac and pulmonary complications are most likely to be associated with poorer prognosis and death. Patients do not generally die from renal failure; cardiopulmonary death or death from stroke is more usual. The syndrome is often accompanied by neurological complications. Patients, although initially conscious, deteriorate rapidly and coma often supervenes.

Pathogenesis

The pathogenesis of this condition, though still obscure, is slowly being unraveled and has received much attention recently. The unique clinical manifestations – small-vessel occlusions leading to multiple organ failure, as opposed to the large venous or arterial thromboses encountered in patients with classic APS – seem to confer a much worse prognosis for CAPS patients. That patients have aPL, often in high titers, makes this a distinct subset of APS.

Molecular mimicry was proposed as an etiologic pathway by Asherson and Shoenfeld.[10] Kitchens has referred to the condition as a 'thrombotic storm', and hypothesized that the vascular occlusions in patients were responsible for the ongoing thrombosis – 'thrombosis begets thrombosis'.[11] Merrill and Asherson recently reviewed evidence that suggests a continuum exists between the several disorders in which localized and diffuse microvascular thromboses lead to similar pathology.[6] These include TTP,[12] hemolytic–uremic syndrome (HUS) in which a relationship to preceding infections with shiga-toxin-producing organisms is seen, thrombotic microangiopathic hemolytic anemia (TMHA) and HELLP syndrome, as well as postpartum renal failure, malignant hypertension, pre-eclampsia and scleroderma renal crisis.

In several of these conditions, similar triggering factors and clinical manifestations have been noted, such as severe thrombocytopenia, microangiopathic hemolytic anemia, fever, renal and neurological complications, and response to plasma exchange.[13] It is interesting that aPL has been reported in many of these conditions, with or without the presence of SLE. The association of aPL with these TMHA-like disorders might, in fact, be stronger than previously appreciated.[14]

The presence of schistocytes in CAPS patients may often blur the differential diagnosis between CAPS and TTP, particularly in those patients predominantly with involvement of the kidneys or central nervous system who also have demonstrable titers of aPL. Several 'overlap' presentations of HELLP syndrome and CAPS have been documented.[15–17]

The role of complement in aPL-induced thrombosis has received much attention recently. Pierangeli et al. stressed the role of complement fractions C3 and C5 in aPL-mediated thrombosis.[18] Work on the role of complement in the etiopathogenesis of fetal loss in murine models by the Salmon group in New York[19] has recently been extended by the group from Harvard University in Boston. Hart et al.[20] and Fleming et al.[21] demonstrated that complement activation plays an important role in both local and remote tissue injury. It is possible that gut barrier dysfunction (e.g. from ischemia induced by small-vessel occlusive disease in CAPS) may lead to bacterial translocation to the lung, with a subsequent increase in complement-mediated neutrophil infiltration due to activation of the lectin complement pathway via ficolins. This research might help to explain some of the odd features of CAPS.

The high frequency of abdominal symptomatology in CAPS patients and the much higher frequency of pulmonary complications such as alveolar hemorrhage lend circumstantial credence to the following clinical scenario:

- complement becomes activated in necrotic bowel tissue
- aPLs are naturally occurring antibodies involved in apoptosis

- a breakdown of the bowel–blood barrier means organisms are carried to lung tissue where complement is activated
- capillary damage ensues, with alveolar hemorrhage mediated via ficolins.

This hypothesis also ties in well with a high frequency of infections, which act as 'triggers' for CAPS.

Treatment

The treatment of CAPS is still associated with 50% mortality and is unsatisfactory. However, it is clear that many patients have not been given the early benefit of the most effective known approaches: repeated plasma exchanges[22] and intravenous immunoglobulins.

High-dose intravenous corticosteroids and parenteral anticoagulants should be the primary therapy, but it is critical to initiate aggressive therapy early in the course of the illness.

Intravenous antibiotics should also be administered if an infection is present or suspected.

Rituximab has been successful in isolated patients with CAPS and severe thrombocytopenia.[23] It has not been attempted in early cases without this complication, but the approach seems reasonable.

New treatments aimed at negating the effects of complement activation will undoubtedly be attempted, and are promising as we become increasingly aware of the importance of complement activation in certain complications of APS such as fetal loss.

Recurrent CAPS

Recurrent CAPS is rare; few cases have been published to date,[24–26] although one patient had 17 relapses.[26] In some patients, relapses were triggered by infections. In others, trauma was responsible (e.g. fracture, cataract surgery) (RA Asherson, personal observations, 2006). However, in the majority, no identifiable precipitating factors were detectable prior to relapse.

There may be a small subset of patients who are prone to relapsing CAPS, possibly because of inherent problems relating to the formation of tissue factor or perhaps genotypic variants of toll-like receptor 4 (TLR4). These possibilities are being explored by the CAPS Survivor Committee in multicenter studies.

Highlights in catastrophic antiphospholipid (Asherson's) syndrome *2005–06*

WHAT'S IN?

- Increased reporting of cases of catastrophic antiphospholipid (Asherson's) syndrome (CAPS) and entry on the website www.med.ub.es/MMMUN/FORUM/CAPS.HTM
- Identification of trigger factors (mainly infection and trauma)
- Recognition that serological disseminated intravascular coagulation (DIC) in some patients can confuse the underlying diagnosis
- Awareness of the relationship between CAPS and underlying infections and the ensuing multiorgan failure, not unlike that observed in non-aPL patients with sepsis
- Awareness of the high frequency of acute respiratory distress syndrome in patients with CAPS
- Recognition that treatment must be early and effective in order to improve survival
- Continuation of treatment with repeated plasma exchanges and intravenous immunoglobulins, if necessary, for several weeks
- Use of rituximab in patients with severe thrombocytopenia
- Possible use of rituximab as acute initial therapy in patients who are unresponsive to more conventional treatment options

WHAT'S OUT?

- Unnecessary delays in the institution of appropriate therapy, with consequent fatal outcome

References

1. Harris EN, Baguley E, Asherson RA et al. Clinical and serological features of the 'antiphospholipid syndrome' (APS). *Br J Rheumatol* 1987;26(suppl 2): 19abstr.

2. Piette JC, Cervera R, Levy RA et al. The catastrophic antiphospholipid syndrome – Asherson's syndrome. *Ann Med Interne (Paris)* 2003;154:195–6.

3. Asherson RA, Cervera R, Merrill JT. The microangiopathic antiphospholipid syndrome (MAPS). A continuum of conditions? *Future Rheumatol* 2006; in press.

4. McCarty GA, Baddour VT, Giesler L et al. Antiphospholipid antibody syndrome (APS) in 227 patients: comparison of IgG/M/LA+ vs. IgA only vs. seronegative APS (SNAPS) Pts. Proc IXth Int Symp on aPL. *J Autoimmun* 2000;15:A78.

5. Marai I, Zandman-Goddard G, Shoenfeld Y. The systemic nature of the antiphospholipid syndrome. *Scand J Rheumatol* 2004;33:365–72.

6. Merrill JT, Asherson RA. Catastrophic antiphospholipid syndrome. *Nat Clin Pract Rheumatol* 2006;2:81–9.

7. Asherson RA. The catastrophic antiphospholipid syndrome. *J Rheumatol* 1992:19:508–12.

8. Bucciarelli S, Espinosa G, Asherson RA et al. The acute respiratory distress syndrome in catastrophic antiphospholipid syndrome: analysis of a series of 47 patients. *Ann Rheum Dis* 2006;.65:81–6.

9. Asherson RA, Espinosa G, Cervera R et al. Disseminated intravascular coagulation in catastrophic antiphospholipid syndrome: clinical and haematological characteristics of 23 patients. *Ann Rheum Dis* 2005;64:943–6.

10. Asherson RA, Shoenfeld Y. The role of infection in the pathogenesis of catastrophic antiphospholipid syndrome – molecular mimicry? *J Rheumatol* 2000;27:12–14.

11. Kitchens CS. Thrombotic storm: when thrombosis begets thrombosis. *Am J Med* 1998;104:381–5.

12. Musa MO, Nounou R, Sahovic E et al. Fulminant thrombotic thrombocytopenic purpura in two patients with systemic lupus erythematosus and phospholipid autoantibodies. *Eur J Haematol* 2000;64:433–5.

13. Roberts G, Gordon MM, Porter D et al. Acute renal failure complicating HELLP syndrome, SLE and anti-phospholipid syndrome; successful outcome using plasma exchange therapy. *Lupus* 2003;12: 251–7.

14. Espinosa G, Bucciarelli S, Cervera R et al. Thrombotic microangiopathic haemolytic anaemia and antiphospholipid antibodies. *Ann Rheum Dis* 2004;63:730–6.

15. Ilbery M, Jones AR, Samson J. Lupus anticoagulant and HELLP syndrome complicated by placental abruption, hepatic, dermal and adrenal infarction. *Aust N Z J Obstet Gynaecol* 1995;35:215–17.

16. Sinha J, Chowdhry I, Sedan S, Barland P. Bone marrow necrosis and refractory HELLP syndrome in a patient with catastrophic antiphospholipid antibody syndrome. *J Rheumatol* 2002;29:195–7.

17. Koenig M, Roy M, Baccot S et al. Thrombotic microangiopathy with liver, gut and bone infarction (catastrophic antiphospholipid syndrome) associated with HELLP syndrome. *Clin Rheumatol* 2005;24:166–8.

18. Pierangeli SS, Girardi G, Vega-Ostertag M et al. Requirement of activation of complement C3 and C5 for antiphospholipid antibody-mediated thrombophilia. *Arthritis Rheum* 2005;52:2120–4.

19. Salmon JE, Girardi G, Holers VM. Activation of complement mediates antiphospholipid antibody-induced pregnancy loss. *Lupus* 2003;12:535–8.

20. Hart ML, Ceonzo KA, Shaffer LA et al. Gastrointestinal ischemia-reperfusion injury is lectin complement pathway dependent without involving C1q. *J Immunol* 2005;174:6373–80.

21. Fleming SD, Egan RP, Chai C et al. Anti-phospholipid antibodies restore mesenteric ischemia/reperfusion-induced injury in complement receptor 2/complement receptor 1-deficient mice. *J Immunol* 2004;173:7055–61.

22. Rock G, Shumak KH, Sutton DM et al. Cryosupernatant as replacement fluid for plasma exchange in thrombotic thrombocytopenic purpura. Members of the Canadian Apheresis Group. *Br J Haematol* 1996;94:383–6.

23. Ehresmann S, Arkfeld D, Shinada S et al. A novel therapeutic approach for catastrophic antiphospholipid syndrome (CAPS) when conventional therapy with anticoagulation and steroids were unsuccessful. *Ann Rheum Dis* 2004;64(suppl 1):abstr FR10278.

24. Undas A, Swadzba J, Undas R, Musial J. Three episodes of acute multiorgan failure in a woman with secondary antiphospholipid syndrome. [Polish] *Pol Arch Med Wewn* 1998;100:556–60.

25. Cerveny KC, Sawitzke AD. Relapsing catastrophic antiphospholipid antibody syndrome: a mimic for thrombotic thrombocytopenic purpura? *Lupus* 1999;8:477–81.

26. Gordon A, McLean CA, Ryan P, Roberts SK. Steroid-responsive catastrophic antiphopholipid syndrome. *J Gastroenterol Hepatol* 2004;19:479–80.

Regulatory T cells and rheumatic diseases

Martin Rynne MB BCh BAO MRCPI MRCP(UK) and John Isaacs PhD FRCP
Musculoskeletal Research Group, School of Clinical Medical Sciences, University of Newcastle upon Tyne, UK

Autoimmune diseases, which arise from a failure of the body's tolerance mechanisms, affect about 5% of the population. In fact, potentially self-reactive T cells are normally present in all individuals, having evaded negative selection (deletion) in the thymus. By 'silencing' these self-reactive T cells, peripheral tolerance mechanisms – such as peripheral deletion of autoreactive cells, anergy induction (hyporesponsiveness to antigen) and control by regulatory T cells (Tregs) – prevent immune pathology. The past decade has seen a resurgence of interest in Tregs, which include transforming growth factor (TGF)β-producing Th3 cells, interleukin (IL)-10-producing Tr1 cells and $CD4^+CD25^+$ T cells. The latter subset, so-called 'natural' Tregs, have been clearly identified in humans and are the focus of this chapter.[1,2]

Naturally occurring Tregs

$CD4^+CD25^+$ T cells constitute 5–10% of the $CD4^+$ T cells in peripheral blood. In humans, regulatory function is predominantly confined to the 1–2% of cells that stain most strongly for CD25 (so called $CD25^{high}$ or $CD25^{bright}$ cells). The transcription factor FoxP3 is critical for the function of these cells, and genetic deficiency in mice or humans results in fatal autoimmunity.[3] Similarly, depletion of this subset results in a variety of organ-specific autoimmune diseases in animal models. Conversely, administration prevents autoimmune disease in lymphopenic mice, and transfer of $CD4^+CD25^+$ T cells into animals with established immunopathology resolves inflammation.[4]

These observations, in which relatively small numbers of natural Tregs can permanently reverse autoimmunity in animal models, have led to extensive study of Tregs in humans, to determine whether similar manipulations may be beneficial in the treatment of immunopathology in autoimmunity, allergy and transplantation.

Identification of natural Tregs. The precise ontogeny of natural Tregs is unclear, and their characterization has been hampered by lack of a lineage-specific marker. Cytotoxic T-lymphocyte-associated protein 4 (CTLA-4) and the glucocorticoid-induced tumor necrosis factor (TNF) receptor (GITR) are shared by activated T cells, and even FoxP3 is not absolutely specific.[5] Conventionally, CD45RO was thought to be acquired following the recognition of self-antigen in the thymus, but recent work points to the existence of CD5RA expressing 'naïve' natural Tregs in peripheral blood.[6] Natural Tregs have also been partitioned into two subsets defined by the integrins $\alpha_4\beta_1$ and $\alpha_4\beta_7$. Both subsets suppress via a contact-dependent mechanism, but appear to differ in downstream immunomodulatory effects.[7] The functionally active isoform of CD44 may also delineate those cells with maximal suppressive activity.[8]

Human $CD4^+CD25^+$ Tregs have been shown to:

- suppress proliferation of T cells[1]
- inhibit monocyte/macrophage activation,[9] proinflammatory cytokine production and antigen-presenting cell (APC) function
- restrain the maturation and antigen-presenting function of dendritic cells.[10]

Suppression requires signaling through the antigen-specific T-cell receptor. In the mouse (and presumably in people), some Tregs remain quiescent, with a lifespan of months, whereas others proliferate extensively, express multiple activation markers and are continuously activated by tissue self-antigens in the periphery.[11] Such a rapid turnover fits with the finding that both their development and maintenance is highly dependent upon co-stimulatory molecules such as CD28 and IL-2.

Murine models of arthritis and Tregs

$CD25^+$ depletion hastens the onset of severe disease in both collagen-induced (CIA) and antigen-induced arthritis (AIA) models.[12,13] In the former, disease progression was markedly slowed when $CD25^+$-depleted mice were infused with sufficient numbers of natural Tregs. The transferred cells were detectable in joint-draining lymph nodes, synovial fluid and inflamed synovial tissue 1–2 days after injection, raising the possibility that natural Tregs control CIA locally via both afferent (priming) and efferent (effector) pathways.[14] Transfer of $CD4^+CD25^+$ cells into immunized mice at the time of induction of AIA also decreased the severity of disease, but was unable to cure established disease.[13] Here, transferred $CD4^+CD25^+$ cells also showed preferential accumulation in the inflamed joint.

Tregs in rheumatoid arthritis

Due to the lack of a specific marker, it has been difficult to definitively enumerate natural Tregs in the inflamed joint. However, several reports attest to an increased frequency in the synovial fluid of patients with rheumatoid arthritis (RA) (and those with other types of inflammatory arthritis), irrespective of disease duration, disease severity, or treatment with disease-modifying antirheumatic drugs.[15–18] In one study, a proportion of natural Tregs from the synovial fluid displayed an activated phenotype with an enhanced suppressive capacity compared with Tregs in the peripheral blood. This was offset, however, by effector T cells (Teffs) in the synovial fluid being more resistant to suppression than their counterparts in the peripheral blood. Thus, although natural Tregs appear to be recruited to inflamed synovium to suppress arthritis, their attempts may be thwarted by the reduced susceptibility of local effector T cells.[19]

A number of studies have reported reduced circulating natural Tregs in a variety of human autoimmune diseases. However, the data in RA vary, with some studies suggesting normal numbers,[15,18,20] others suggesting an increase[19] and others reporting a reduction.[16,21] At least some of this variability is attributable to differences in disease stage and therapy, but there is also a variability in the phenotypic definition of natural Tregs between studies. In one study, circulating $CD4^+CD25^{high}$ T cells in patients with RA were functionally defective and unable to suppress Teffs in peripheral blood.[20] These data are consistent with those reported in multiple sclerosis,[22] but differ from the findings in synovial fluid.[19] Three months of anti-TNFα therapy (infliximab) restored the suppressive capacity of natural Tregs, with responders demonstrating a higher frequency of circulating $CD4^+CD25^{high}$ T cells after treatment than before.[20] Adalimumab was also found to increase numbers and improve function of natural Tregs in peripheral blood at 15 days. Although Treg numbers had fallen by 6 months, they remained higher than pretreatment levels.[23] One simple interpretation of these data is that natural Tregs travel to the inflamed synovium from peripheral blood and return once inflammation is controlled. In addition, however, TNFα blockade may exert important immunoregulatory effects in addition to its potent anti-inflammatory activities.

Tregs in juvenile idiopathic arthritis

Patients with persistent oligoarticular juvenile idiopathic arthritis (JIA) (which often carries a relatively benign, self-remitting course) displayed significantly higher frequencies of circulating $CD4^+CD25^{bright}$ T cells than their counterparts with extended oligoarticular JIA who have a poor prognosis.[24] There were also more $FoxP3^+CD4^+CD25^+$ T cells in the synovial fluid, suggesting that the progression of extended oligoarticular JIA may be related to a failure of $CD4^+CD25^+$ T cells to either home towards or expand at the site of inflammation. Recently, CD27 has been shown to distinguish natural Tregs from activated/effector T cells in the synovial fluid of patients with JIA. Synovial-fluid cells were again shown to be more potent than their circulating counterparts.[25]

Autologous stem-cell transplantation has provided excellent benefit in children with otherwise refractory JIA. Published series suggest that 50% of children enter long-term full remission, while an additional significant proportion gain partial remission and response to previously inadequate therapies. Recent data link these good outcomes with the appearance of natural Tregs in peripheral blood.[26] Prior to therapy there were proportionally fewer natural Tregs in blood than in age-matched controls. After therapy there

Highlights in **regulatory T cells and rheumatic diseases** *2005–06*

WHAT'S IN?

- Lymphocyte-mediated suppression
- Cells as therapeutic agents
- Therapeutic tolerance induction

WHAT'S OUT?

- The concept that autoimmunity is necessarily a lifelong affliction

WHAT'S NEEDED?

- Robust markers of natural T regulatory cells
- Biomarkers of tolerance induction

was an initial lymphopenia-induced homeostatic proliferation of Tregs followed by the appearance of circulating naive Tregs, consistent with de-novo thymic output. These exciting data suggest that it is possible to restore powerful peripheral tolerance mechanisms in at least some human autoimmune diseases.

Natural Tregs as therapeutic agents

Natural Tregs can be expanded in vitro by stimulation with a combination of anti-CD3 and anti-CD28 monoclonal antibodies (mAbs), along with high doses of IL-2. Whilst such expanded cells have therapeutic effects in animal models of autoimmunity, their potency is increased many times over if expansion utilizes an autoantigen-specific stimulus. This presumably ensures that their suppressive efforts are focused on the target organ, and should also reduce the likelihood of non-specific immunosuppressive effects.[27]

The ex-vivo expansion of cells raises practical and technical difficulties, although these are not insurmountable. Recently, however, a novel immunomodulatory therapy has been associated with an apparent in-vivo expansion of natural Tregs. In two separate studies, non-mitogenic anti-CD3 mAbs were used to treat patients with recent-onset type 1 diabetes mellitus.[28,29] In both studies, a brief course of therapy was associated with stabilization of clinical status and reduction or reversal of insulin requirements for up to 18 months. In one of these studies, therapy was associated with the appearance of cells with regulatory potential in the peripheral blood. Some of these were IL-10-expressing $CD4^+$ T cells but some were cells with a $CD8^+CD25^{high}FoxP3^+$ phenotype, a potentially novel subset of Tregs.[30,31] Equivalent experiments in mice also suggest that non-mitogenic anti-CD3 monoclonal antibodies lead to the appearance of regulatory T cells, in this case expressing TGFβ.[32]

Conclusion

Although in its infancy, the clinical application of Tregs has the potential to introduce a novel treatment paradigm into the field of rheumatology. The administration of ex-vivo expanded antigen-specific Tregs, 'resetting' of the autoreactive immune system using high-dose chemotherapy followed by autologous stem cells (see page 74), or the use of agents such as non-mitogenic anti-CD3 mAbs to induce the cells in vivo, are all applications with the potential to provide long-term benefit from brief interventions.

References

1. Piccirillo CA, Shevach EM. Naturally-occurring $CD4^+CD25^+$ immunoregulatory T cells: central players in the arena of peripheral tolerance. *Semin Immunol* 2004;16:81–8.
2. Ng WF, Duggan PJ, Ponchel F et al. Human CD4(+)CD25(+) cells: a naturally occurring population of regulatory T cells. *Blood* 2001; 98:2736–44.

3. Hori S, Nomura T, Sakaguchi S. Control of regulatory T cell development by the transcription factor Foxp3. *Science* 2003;299: 1057–61.

4. Mottet C, Uhlig HH, Powrie F. Cutting edge: cure of colitis by $CD4^+CD25^+$ regulatory T cells. *J Immunol* 2003;170:3939–43.

5. Roncador G, Brown PJ, Maestre L et al. Analysis of FOXP3 protein expression in human $CD4^+CD25^+$ regulatory T cells at the single-cell level. *Eur J Immunol* 2005; 35: 1681–91.

6. Seddiki N, Santner-Nanan B, Tangye SG et al. Persistence of naive $CD45RA^+$ regulatory T cells in adult life. *Blood* 2005 Dec 6; [Epub ahead of print].

7. Stassen M, Fondel S, Bopp T et al. Human $CD25^+$ regulatory T cells: two subsets defined by the integrins $\alpha_4\beta_7$ or $\alpha_4\beta_1$ confer distinct suppressive properties upon $CD4^+$ T helper cells. *Eur J Immunol* 2004;34:1303–11.

8. Firan M, Dhillon S, Estess P, Siegelman MH. Suppressor activity and potency among regulatory T cells is discriminated by functionally active CD44. *Blood* 2006;107:619–27.

9. Taams LS, van Amelsfort JMR, Tiemessen MM et al. Modulation of monocyte/macrophage function by human $CD4^+CD25^+$ regulatory T cells. *Human Immunol* 2005; 66:222–30.

10. Misra N, Bayry J, Lacroix-Desmazes S et al. Cutting edge: human $CD4^+CD25^+$ T cells restrain the maturation and antigen-presenting function of dendritic cells. *J Immunol* 2004;172:4676–80.

11. Fisson S, Darrasse-Jeze G, Litvinova E et al. Continuous activation of autoreactive $CD4^+$ $CD25^+$ regulatory T cells in the steady state. *J Exp Med* 2003;198: 737–46.

12. Morgan ME, Sutmuller RPM, Witteveen HJ et al. $CD25^+$ cell depletion hastens the onset of severe disease in collagen-induced arthritis. *Arthritis Rheum* 2003;48:1452–60.

13. Frey O, Petrow PK, Gajda M et al. The role of regulatory T cells in antigen-induced arthritis: aggravation of arthritis after depletion and amelioration after transfer of $CD4^+CD25^+$ T cells. *Arthritis Res Ther* 2005;7:R291–301.

14. Morgan ME, Flierman R, van Duivenvoorde LM et al. Effective treatment of collagen-induced arthritis by adoptive transfer of $CD25^+$ regulatory T cells. *Arthritis Rheum* 2005;52:2212–21.

15. Cao D, Malmström V, Baecher-Allan C et al. Isolation and functional characterization of regulatory $CD25brightCD4^+$ T cells from the target organ of patients with rheumatoid arthritis. *Eur J Immunol* 2003;33:215–23.

16. Cao D, van Vollenhoven R, Klareskog L et al. CD25brightCD4$^+$ regulatory T cells are enriched in inflamed joints of patients with chronic rheumatic disease. *Arthritis Res Ther* 2004;6:R335–46.

17. Liu MF, Wang CR, Fung LL et al. The presence of cytokine-suppressive CD4$^+$CD25$^+$ T cells in the peripheral blood and synovial fluid of patients with rheumatoid arthritis. *Scand J Immunol* 2005;62:312–17.

18. Mottonen M, Heikkinen J, Mustonen L et al. CD4$^+$ CD25$^+$ T cells with the phenotypic and functional characteristics of regulatory T cells are enriched in the synovial fluid of patients with rheumatoid arthritis. *Clin Exp Immunol* 2005;140:360–7.

19. van Amelsfort JM, Jacobs KM, Bijlsma JW et al. CD4($^+$)CD25($^+$) regulatory T cells in rheumatoid arthritis: differences in the presence, phenotype, and function between peripheral blood and synovial fluid. *Arthritis Rheum* 2004;50:2775–85.

20. Ehrenstein MR, Evans JG, Singh A et al. Compromised function of regulatory T cells in rheumatoid arthritis and reversal by anti TNFalpha therapy. *J Exp Med* 2004;200:277–85.

21. Lawson CA, Brown AK, Bejarano V et al. Early rheumatoid arthritis is associated with a deficit in the CD4$^+$CD25^{high} regulatory T-cell population in peripheral blood. *Rheumatology (Oxford)* 2006; in press.

22. Baecher-Allan C, Brown JA, Freeman GJ, Hafler DA. CD4$^+$ CD25^{high} regulatory cells in human peripheral blood. *J Immunol* 2001;167:1245–53.

23. Vigna-Pérez M, Abud-Mendoza C, Portillo-Salazar H et al. Immune effects of therapy with adalimumab in patients with rheumatoid arthritis. *Clin Exp Immunol* 2005;141:372–80.

24. de Kleer IM, Wedderburn LR, Taams LS et al. CD4$^+$CD25bright regulatory T cells actively regulate inflammation in the joints of patients with the remitting form of juvenile idiopathic arthritis. *J Immunol* 2004;172:6435–43.

25. Ruprecht CR, Gattorno M, Ferlito F et al. Coexpression of CD25 and CD27 identifies FoxP3$^+$ regulatory T cells in inflamed synovia. *J Exp Med* 2005;201: 1793–803.

26. de Kleer I, Vastert B, Klein M et al. Autologous stem cell transplantation for autoimmunity induces immunologic self-tolerance by reprogramming autoreactive T-cells and restoring the CD4$^+$CD25$^+$ immune regulatory network. *Blood* 2006;107:1696–702.

27. Tang Q, Henriksen KJ, Bi M et al. In vitro-expanded antigen-specific regulatory T cells suppress autoimmune diabetes. *J Exp Med* 2004;199:1455–65.

28. Herold KC, Hagopian W, Auger JA et al. Anti-CD3 monoclonal antibody in new-onset type 1 diabetes mellitus. *N Engl J Med* 2002;346:1692–8.

29. Keymeulen B, Vandemeulebroucke E, Ziegler AG et al. Insulin needs after CD3-antibody therapy in new-onset type 1 diabetes. *N Engl J Med* 2005;352:2598–608.

30. Herold KC, Burton JB, Francois F et al. Activation of human T cells by FcR nonbinding anti-CD3 mAb, hOKT3gamma1(Ala-Ala). *J Clin Invest* 2003;111:409–18.

31. Bisikirska B, Colgan J, Luban J et al. TCR stimulation with modified anti-CD3 mAb expands $CD8^+$ T cell population and induces $CD8^+CD25^+$ Tregs. *J Clin Invest* 2005;115: 2904–13.

32. Chatenoud L. CD3-specific antibody-induced active tolerance: from bench to bedside. *Nat Rev Immunol* 2003;3:123–32.

Other titles from Health Press that might interest you...

Do you already know about *Patient Pictures*, our series designed to help healthcare professionals explain disorders and treatments to their patients?

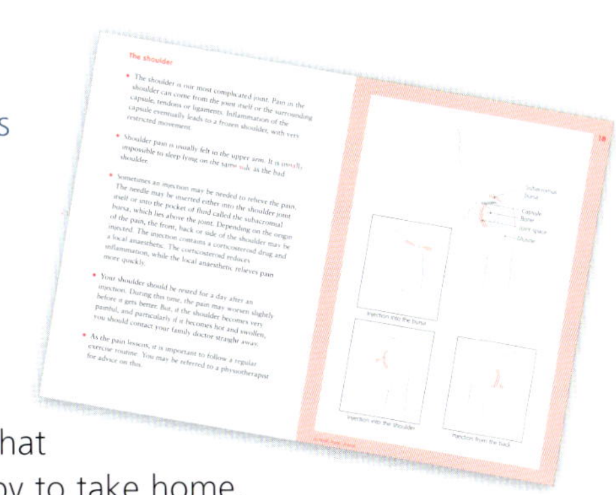

- Double-page spreads dedicated to the topics you need to explain
- Each spread clearly illustrated and supplemented with simple text
- Spreads designed to stand alone so that you can give your patient a photocopy to take home.

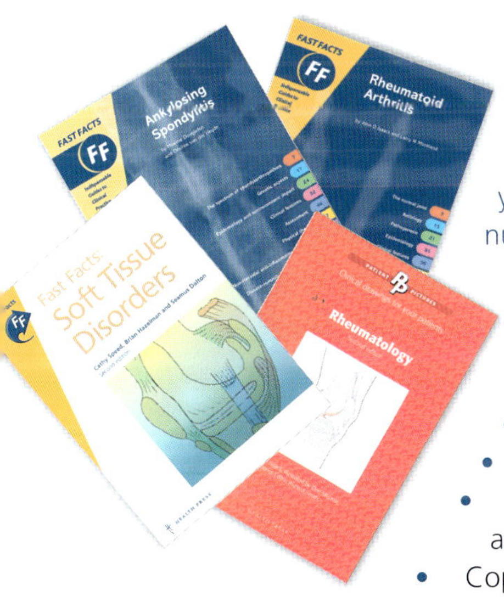

We also publish *Fast Facts*, the ultimate medical handbook series. If you are a primary care physician, a nurse, a student or a specialist reading outside your field, these books are for you.

- Written by world experts
- Concise and practical
- Up to date
- Designed for ease of reading and reference
- Copiously illustrated with useful photographs, diagrams and charts

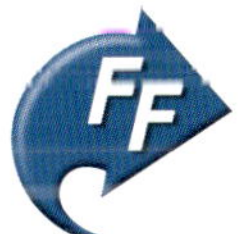

Imagine if every time you wanted to know something you knew where to look...

Orders

To order via the website, or to find regional distributors, please go to www.fastfacts.com

For telephone orders, please call +44 (0)1752 202301 (Europe), 1 800 247 6553 (USA, toll free) or +1 419 281 1802 (Americas)